Recalled to Health

Free Yourself from a Self-Imposed Prison of Bad Habits

Tim Hennessy, M.D.

T0273398

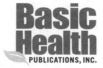

Basic Health
PUBLICATIONS, INC.

The information contained in this book is based upon the research and personal and professional experiences of the authors. It is not intended as a substitute for consulting with your physician or other healthcare provider. Any attempt to diagnose and treat an illness should be done under the direction of a healthcare professional.

The publisher does not advocate the use of any particular healthcare protocol but believes the information in this book should be available to the public. The publisher and authors are not responsible for any adverse effects or consequences resulting from the use of the suggestions, preparations, or procedures discussed in this book. Should the reader have any questions concerning the appropriateness of any procedures or preparation mentioned, the authors and the publisher strongly suggest consulting a professional healthcare advisor.

Basic Health Publications, Inc.
28812 Top of the World Drive
Laguna Beach, CA 92651
949-715-7327 • www.basichealthpub.com

Library of Congress Cataloging-in-Publication Data

Hennessy, Tim
   Recalled to health / Tim Hennessy.
     p. cm.
   Includes bibliographical references and index.
   ISBN 978-1-59120-257-8
   1. Health behavior. 2. Health—Psychological aspects. 3. Lifestyles—
Health aspects. I. Title.
   RA776.9.H46   2009
   613—dc22
                                                            2009021240

Editor: Roberta W. Waddell
Typesetting/Book design: Gary A. Rosenberg
Cover design: Mike Stromberg

Printed in the United States of America

10   9   8   7   6   5   4   3   2   1

CONTENTS

This book is dedicated to
Mary, May, Thomas, and Lizzy.
My best of times are when I'm with you.

ACKNOWLEDGMENTS

It was his wristband I noticed first. It said, "READ," so I began talking books with him. This is how I met my agent, and this is where I need to start my acknowledgments. I owe a debt of gratitude to many people for helping me with this project, but none are more deserving than my agent, Stanley Budner. Your help has made all the difference, Stan. Thank you.

I also have to give a special thank you to my editor, Bobby Waddell. Your efforts helped to make my work shine, and from your efforts I learned a great deal. Thank you, too.

With writing, there is always a point when you have to show your work to someone outside your immediate circle of family and friends, someone outside your comfort zone. For *Recalled to Health*, this moment came when the University of Delaware graciously offered to review it. I can't thank Dr. Donald Mell (English professor) and Karen Druliner (editor) enough for all their assistance and due diligence in critically evaluating this piece, making it worthy to submit to publishers.

As for friends, there are many to whom I am grateful, but in particular I have to thank Bob Pasquale, Alisa Bowman, Bob Catalano, and Damian Demnicki. Together, your support has been outstanding, your advice has been on the mark, and your confidence in me motivational. Thank you all.

As you will soon read, many of my stories are homegrown, straight from experiences dealing with my mom and dad. As someone once said, they *didn't tell me how to live, they lived, and let me watch them do it.*

Lastly, and most importantly, I have to thank my wife, Mary, without whom this book wouldn't even have been attempted. You have always been my inspiration. I am lucky to have you as my wife, and this book is for you.

INTRODUCTION

In a word, this book is about *freedom*. It is intended to promote your freedom by inspiring you to live healthier. In the process, it is hoped that you will become less dependent on our flawed healthcare system, less dependent on medications, and more emboldened to live life to its fullest, unrestrained by the physical constraints of poor health. For some of you, this book will help to maintain your health. For others, it will help reclaim it. In either case, it will help to strengthen your mind, so you can strengthen your body.

The focus of this book, and my reason for writing it, is to create a medical foundation for you that will give you a better understanding of medical topics, and will, in turn, empower you to take charge of your own health. Cholesterol, blood pressure, diet and weight management, exercise, sleeping habits, and the role of nature in health are some of the topics discussed in full here, along with suggestions for optimum actions, behaviors, or treatments. The chapters all end with a helpful summary of tips; the back of the book has numerous References, fully cited and listed by chapters; and there is a full Index.

Medicine—The Best and Worst of Times

A Tale of Two Cities, Charles Dickens' inspiring story, opens with the classic line, "These were the best of times, these were the worst of times." He was talking about the political and social life of Europe in the late eighteenth century, with a particular emphasis on the French Revolution. At the beginning, he related a cryptic message about someone being *recalled to life* after having been unjustly jailed in the Bastille for seventeen years.

It is not difficult to draw parallels to that phrase when discussing medicine in this time, an age of extraordinary medical advancements overall. On the plus side, the best of times include a technology that is unprecedented in its ability to help establish an accurate diagnosis; newer medicines continually being developed that are offering reasons for hope where there were none; and physicians who are increasing their skills by refining them and narrowing their scope, becoming more specialized in the process. The result of all this is seemingly unlimited potential for the world of medicine to help as never before.

Yet with all these advancements, there come many problems, which is where the other half of Dickens' sentence about the worst of times comes into play. Those problems include a fairly significant portion of society that still has a limited access to medical care, and an even larger percentage that is worrying about how they are going to pay for the new technology, the new medicines, and the more specialized physicians. When factoring in the additional frustrations of dealing with the seemingly endless bureaucracy of health insurance companies, it is easy to see why people are not as happy about the advances as they could be.

These contrasts are even greater if you look at the realm of personal healthcare. Because of all the medical advances, people are actually living longer. The Centers for Disease Control and Prevention (CDC) report that the average life expectancy for men rose to 74.4 years in 2001, representing an incredible three-year increase compared to ten years earlier. And the death rates for the three perpetually leading causes of death—cancer, heart disease, and strokes—were found to consistently decline during this same time period. More people are exercising. More people are watching their diets.

Yet, taken as a whole, society appears to be *less* healthy. As a nation, Americans are gaining weight in record numbers. According to the National Health and Nutrition Examination Survey (NHANES), over 64 percent of Americans, roughly two out of every three adults, were considered overweight in the year 2000. Approximately 31 percent of the population, 59 million people, were considered outright obese.

With this weight gain, the expected impact on diabetes and hypertension naturally followed. The CDC reported that, during the 1990s alone, the incidence of diabetes increased from 5.1 percent to 7.3 percent and that of hypertension rose from 28 percent to 33 percent. More people are depressed. More people are anxious. And more people are feeling stressed than ever before.

Ultimately, people do not seem as happy as they should be, given the relative prosperity of the time. In many ways, this discontent seems to arise from not developing good habits—habits that represent the cornerstone of healthier living, and center on maintaining discipline about the small things in life.

If you can change the manner in which you do these small things, the ripples from this action can lead to a fairly large wave. The small changes can lead to lasting life-improving and life-prolonging results. In essence, small investments can pay huge dividends.

Paraphrasing Charles Dickens' words about the man recalled to life from his lengthy prison sentence, I am writing about how people can be recalled to health, drawing on the inspiration I receive from many of my patients to hopefully inspire you in your efforts to change. I also hope to provide a framework that can serve as a practical guide to help you get started. In sum, I want to help you free yourself from a self-imposed jail of bad habits and be *Recalled to Health*.

1

Starting Point— Wanting to Be Healthy

My wealth is health and perfect ease.
—Sir Edward Dyer, *My Mind to Me a Kingdom Is*

"Your health is your most valuable asset." I can still hear my high school gym teacher saying those words twenty years ago. It was true then, it is true now, and it will always be true. Every time I have been sick, with even the most minor of illnesses, I'd think what I wouldn't give to be feeling better. Your health is your most taken-for-granted asset, and it's something that isn't truly valued until it has gone away.

Recently, a patient came to my office at his wife's urging. He was a thirty-year-old man with no previous medical problems. Married for three years, he was was the proud father of a six-month baby girl. Generally he reported feeling well, except that, over the past year, since before the baby had been born, he was more tired than usual. He felt stressed at work, but nothing out of the ordinary for him. He didn't feel depressed. Basically, he didn't know why he felt so bad. Tired of hearing him complain, his wife insisted he make an appointment. Immediately, he and I both noticed the significant increase in his weight. Prior to his marriage, he was a respectable, slightly overweight, 215 pounds. At the time of this visit, he thought his weight might have gone up a little, but was shocked to see he had actually gained *forty-five* pounds. He attributed this weight gain to a variety of factors. With the arrival of the new baby, he was no longer exercising, he was eating a lot more fast food at work, and he was also eating larger portions of food at every meal.

His exam was relatively normal except for the fact that his blood pressure was slightly elevated at 148 over 92. Lab tests prefatory to the visit showed that he had an elevated blood sugar, 118 milligrams, which meant he was bordering on type 2 diabetes. To make matters worse, his cholesterol was also elevated at greater than 300 milligrams. Needless to say, he was upset by these findings, and even more upset when I started talking about the potential medications he might need to treat his hypertension, elevated cholesterol, and borderline diabetes.

He was definitely not interested in taking medications for the rest of his life, and instead chose to make some changes in his behavior. Without my telling him, he realized that his fatigue was secondary to his new sedentary lifestyle and parallel weight gain. Convinced he could fix these problems on his own, he asked for six months to get himself into shape. Having heard these promises before, I doubted he would be able to change, but was certainly willing to let him try. When six months passed and he came back for his follow-up appointment, there was a big smile on his face. He was a new person, feeling better than he had in years. He returned with thirty pounds less on his frame, and as a result, his repeat blood work showed that his blood sugar had returned to normal, his cholesterol had dropped over sixty points, and his blood pressure was no longer elevated. He told a truly inspiring tale.

Immediately after his initial appointment, he made a conscious decision to begin taking control of his life. He focused on nutrition at every meal. He stopped eating junk food, began reading labels, and started exercising again. At the outset, he had only been able to walk a few blocks before he had to stop. Not willing to be defeated, he continued trying until he was able to walk two miles without stopping. Then he started jogging on the local high school track, at first going only short distances before having to walk again. He continued this walking and jogging pattern, until he was able to run the whole time, increasing his distance each and every time he went to run. The end result was that he felt great, his numbers improved significantly, and he avoided the label of diabetes with all its negative connotations. He also avoided the addition of at least two or three new medications, which would likely have been permanent.

The most important point of this story, though, is not that he changed, but *why* he changed, what motivated him to fix his problems. It wasn't a desire all of a sudden to live healthier, though that was the end result; it wasn't a desire to do whatever it takes to feel better, though that is definitely what he wanted; it wasn't even a desire to please his wife or doctor, though that was what we wanted. The driving force behind his behavior, the real reason he changed, was that *he didn't want to take medications.* The thought scared him to the point that he was ready to take action.

Each of you has an underwritten set of rules governing your behavior. When these rules get threatened, as the no-medication mindset of my patient had been, the desire to change becomes very strong. It is my hope, through writing this book, that I can help you develop your set of rules, and in the process, inspire you onward to a healthier, happier life.

Health—Gone Away

Primary care physicians talk to people every day when their health has *gone away.* It is at this point that people begin equating health with value and become willing to do almost anything to get back their lost asset. The real challenge is to keep this connection between health and value at the forefront of consciousness. This is a very difficult thing to do. Everyone wants to be healthy. Everyone knows it is good to be healthy, though not everyone thinks about their health on a daily basis. In fact, only a small percentage of people seem to have mastered this connection, and in so doing, they have discovered one of the major secrets to living a fulfilling and happy life. Every day, these people make choices in the small things that are in keeping with their overall plan of good health. They make good choices regarding their diet and the amount of sleep that they get. They keep their weight in check and their stress level under control. They always make exercise a true priority on a daily basis. This is the group you want to be in because, as might be expected, there is another group of people on the extreme opposite end of the spectrum who *never* think about their health, with predictably negative outcomes, and that's not a place you want to be.

These people place little value on trying to be healthy, and they rarely contemplate changing behaviors to improve themselves. Usually, they only make appointments to see their doctors when they are very sick. They don't believe in routine checkups, or preventive health measures. They focus all their energies on the here and now, and their approach is way too shortsighted. By following this *carpe diem* approach, they are sacrificing much of their future happiness. They could be avoiding a world of pain, both for them and their family, by simply making a few behavioral changes. What they, and most people, don't realize is that these changes are well within their reach. In terms of energy expenditure, the difference between the two approaches to life is not that great—the healthy approach is within the realm of everyone if they so choose.

The *health conscious* and the *health unconscious* represent only small portions of the total population, however—the two ends of a traditional bell curve. Most people fall somewhere in the middle. A couple of times a year, some sort of trigger elevates health to a priority wherein it is actively sought. Often, it is something as simple as a shirt not fitting or a comment taken out of context. Just as January finds a president preparing the State of the Union address in which he describes where the nation is, where it is going, and how it is going to get there, people are doing the same on an individual basis. Unfortunately, the resolutions rarely make it past the end of January. The central theme persists—the inability to keep health issues at the top of the mental daily planner.

Health Is Wealth

Why is health valuable? It seems like a simple question, which could be answered easily, yet few people ever actually take the time to think about it. Ultimately, being healthy is a way for people to maximize their freedom to do as they please. Being healthy is being free. Being free is being happy. Before he wrote the Declaration of Independence, Thomas Jefferson had extensively studied many of the great philosophers of the Renaissance, who had contemplated the ultimate meaning of life and how people could make the most of the opportunity given to them. Building on their writings, Jefferson eloquently inserted into the document his timeless words about the basic "inalienable rights" of all men that included the right to "life, liberty, and the pursuit of happiness." Without health, however, people would have great difficulty exercising these basic rights. It is the glue that holds them together. The healthier a person is, the greater the quality of life, the larger the scope of freedom, and the more aggressive the pursuit of happiness can be.

Health is, in many ways, comparable to a type of currency, affording people the opportunity to live as they see fit. The better their health, the more currency they have to pursue self-interests. Activities, such as golf and travel, become more commonplace, work becomes more productive, and relationships become more secure when people are healthy. Often forgotten, though, is how this health currency can be spent on others. Spending more time with children and grandchildren, helping neighbors when they need a hand, and visiting friends when they need someone to lean on, all are easier to do when you are in good health. These activities, more than anything else, are at the foundation of a happy, fulfilled life.

What If—Exploring What Could Have Been

There is an extremely interesting history book, edited by Robert Cowley, entitled *What If.* It is a collection of essays, written mostly by military historians, that explore the world of so-called counterfactual history—history that didn't happen but very easily could have. As an example, there has always been rampant speculation, some call it second-guessing, as to what may have happened in World War II if Hitler hadn't invaded Russia. Many are able to give convincing arguments that the eventual outcome of the war may have been drastically different, if not for that one decision, and the world's citizens may all have had to end up learning the Nazi salute.

When taking care of their patients with multiple medical problems, physicians sometime delve into the world of counterfactual medical history. They wonder if people were just fated to get certain problems based on their genetics, or whether there had been a crossroads in their life when they should have gone left instead of right. As is often the case, the answer probably lies somewhere in the middle. Undeniably, genetics strongly influence the medical problems that may arise in an individual. But, a person's choices, with regard to healthy and unhealthy behaviors, also play a vital role. By changing one decision, the outcome of a major war may have been reversed; by changing one behavior, potential medical problems might easily be averted.

For example, even if you have a strong family history of heart disease, it is very possible to take steps earlier in life to literally change the future. Hypertension, diabetes, and elevated cholesterol are well-known risk factors for the development of premature heart disease in many people. The simple step of controlling your weight can help you modify these risk factors by reducing your blood pressure, reducing your likelihood of developing diabetes, and lowering your cholesterol numbers. By doing this, you would have significantly reduced your chances of getting early heart disease. This one decision of carefully watching your weight can lead to immeasurable benefits for you and your family.

There are many other small decisions you can make to also prevent heart attacks, such as quitting smoking, remembering to take a daily aspirin, or possibly, as a last resort, taking medications to help modify the aforementioned risk factors. The point here, as I said, is that small changes can lead to big results.

Unfortunately, people do not have the ability to look into the future to see the medical problems they may be averting. As a result, it is difficult to appreciate the value of these small changes. For this reason, it is important for you to have some understanding of the science and the studies behind your physician's recommendations in order to better appreciate the value these changes might bring.

Being Recalled—The Ongoing Story

If his story were a Hollywood movie, my patient's struggle, which opened this chapter, would end with him running on the track. He would be smiling and looking great. The music from *Chariots of Fire* would be playing, the credits would be rolling, and the audience would be leaving the theater feeling good about what they had just seen. But, alas, his struggle didn't end there, it didn't end when he accomplished his goal; in fact, in many ways, it was only getting started.

I recently saw his wife in the office for her routine checkup. Several years had elapsed since her husband's remarkable transformation. But, unfortunately, she told a story that doctors have heard before. Her husband did well for the first six to nine months, she proudly reported, but then life started getting in the way. His work became more demanding, his baby, now a toddler, needed more of his time, and his house projects started piling up on him. As a result, his exercise routine was continually disrupted until, finally, it ended, and his old habits began to reappear. The tiredness returned, and so, too, did his lost weight. His wife, worried about him, did what a good wife does, and made him a doctor's appointment without telling him.

When he came in for his visit, he had a sheepish look on his face, much like a kid being called to a principal's office. His weight was up twenty pounds, not good, but better than the forty-five pounds he had gained before, we both rationalized; his blood pressure was up slightly, and so, too, was his blood sugar. He echoed his desire for no medications, and again asked for six months to improve his numbers. I gave him the six months.

The concept of being recalled is not about suddenly seeing the light, as my patient had done when he was first threatened with serious health problems. It's about remembering the value of following healthy behaviors before the problems arise; it's about setting limits that, when threatened, trigger behavior change; it's about getting organized so preventive healthcare can always have a chance to work; it's about seeing your doctor before you get sick; and it's about doing whatever is needed to get yourself *Recalled to Health*.

2

HABIT'S ROLE IN HEALTH

What reason weaves, by passion is undone . . .
On life's vast ocean diversely we sail,
Reason the card, but passion the gales. . .
—ALEXANDER POPE, *AN ESSAY ON MAN*

I first set foot on a golf course when I was sixteen years old. My dad was entered in a tournament and needed another person to complete his foursome. Considering myself fairly athletic, I thought I could surely compete with a bunch of old guys. Well, needless to say, I was wrong. During the game, I lost close to a dozen golf balls, there were several holes I didn't even bother finishing, and I frequently lost count of how many strokes were taken because I had taken so many strokes. I did win a trophy that day for "Worst in Tournament." If you're going to be bad, be really bad became my face-saving mantra.

After taking a good amount of ribbing from my dad, I was determined I would do better. But, to my surprise, despite practicing every day, reading golf books, and listening to my dad's advice, I improved only marginally. I soon came to realize that the golf swing is a very difficult swing to master. It involves a whole series of unnatural body contortions that must be coordinated into one graceful motion. This motion must be done while simultaneously focusing on a little white ball. For best results, the ball needs to be struck perfectly with the *sweet spot* of the club. It can be, and often is, an absolute nightmare.

For beginners, it is made even more difficult by everyone giving advice . . . "You're bending your knees too much, your stance is all

13

wrong, you have to slow down your club speed," one would say. "Keep your head down, you're not following all the way through with your swing, don't swing so hard," another would interject. As a result, when it's time to take a turn at the tee, usually in front of at least three other golfers (though the first hole may have twenty or more), all those nuggets of advice get repeated over and over in your head.

It's easy to visualize what usually happens. For me, the result was either missing the ball completely, which wasn't too bad because you could pass it off as a practice swing, or mis-hitting the ball, which was worse because you have to repeat the whole process only a few feet from where you had started. When you go up to the ball thinking too much, it almost never works out well. The secret is to work on one aspect of the swing at a time, and practice that one aspect until it becomes natural, a part of the subconscious. Then you start working on other portions of the swing until it all comes together.

Developing Good Health Habits

How do poor golfing skills apply to your health? The keys to developing good habits for better health are similar to the keys for developing a better golf swing.

- They both require learning what should be done, especially at the beginning, in order to avoid having bad habits take root.

- They both require practicing single acts until they become natural and comfortable, before going on to attain bigger goals.

- They both require expanding on what has already been learned—this is what separates those who will improve from those who will not.

- And, they both require understanding that bad shots, and bad days, are going to happen.

Both the good golfer and the healthy person will not let minor setbacks ruin the game, or the overall plan for good health.

Learning the golf swing and learning to change behavior are two very difficult things to do. They require extraordinary patience and determination. They are not short-term projects. Rather, they take time in order to develop and take hold. When new golfers get motivated to improve, they usually direct all their energies toward that goal and literally get consumed with talking about golf, reading about golf, and dreaming about golf. They typically buy a new set of clubs, the best available, make sure they have the right clothes and the proper shoes, basically getting whatever helps them with their game.

Each January, when the majority of people get motivated to be healthier, they, too, direct all their energies toward achieving this goal. They talk about their health and exercise programs to anyone who will listen. They buy nutrition books and exercise equipment—the treadmill is especially popular. They spend much of their days thinking about how enlightened they have become, almost pitying their uninformed, out-of-shape friends and co-workers. Then, what usually happens? Just as the new golfer starts getting frustrated by the lack of appreciable results, the same thing happens to the person who is trying to be healthier. The lack of immediate results seriously slows the momentum and impetus for change. Gradually, the old familiar habits return, the passion for change is extinguished, and the treadmill serves as an expensive clothes holder.

Changing behavior temporarily is easy; changing behavior for the long term is very, very difficult. Frankly, this is the key to all self-improvement whether you're talking about health, finances, or relationships. Normally, when people get inspired, they get *really* inspired. They introduce multiple changes simultaneously in an effort to address the multiple deficiencies that have become painfully obvious to them. In trying to lose weight, for example, they become so determined that they radically change all aspects of their diet. They cut down calories, cut out junk food, eliminate the snacking, and skip meals. They become the golfer thinking of five things at once as they walk up to the tee. But, they are going to fail, and as a result, will feel miserable about themselves.

This is a process that repeats itself at least a couple times a year. These recurrent mini-failures definitely start taking their toll. They gradually erode confidence, lessen self-esteem, and take away determination. The result is that they stop trying to improve and fall into the realm of the health-unconscious.

Getting Inspired

In physics, there is a concept known as the Law of Perpetual Motion. Basically, it states that a moving object will continue going in the same direction, unless it is acted upon by other forces.

In much the same way, people's behavior imitates this concept by going in the same direction, unless it, too, is forced to change by other factors. These factors, although varying in terms of how much and how long they affect behavior, are similar in that they cause people to react. Understanding these factors, or triggers for change, will help gain a better understanding of what really inspires people; what really motivates them to improve.

The most basic of these triggers, and the one most influential in the short term, is reacting to how you are feeling. If you are not feeling well, if you are in pain or are uncomfortable, then it is very likely you will makes some changes to start feeling better. Everybody exhibits this pattern of behaving, even those who don't otherwise care about their health.

Even though reacting to how you feel is the strongest of all the triggers, it is also the least sustaining. Once you're feeling better, the impetus for change will be gone, and too often you will return to your previous pattern of living.

Another very common trigger for change is reacting to numbers, objective measures indicating how your health may be doing. Whether it is your weight, your blood-pressure reading, your lab results, or your dress size, many people tend to react, or overreact, to numbers, and try to improve them faster than is realistically possible. This trigger that starts out strong in its likelihood to promote change, usually loses its effectiveness once the numbers start getting forgotten, which is often in only a few days. The main problem with this trigger is that many people don't look at numbers that frequently, and, as a result, don't give themselves the opportunity to adjust their behavior in order to right that which may be wrong.

People also use the calendar as a trigger for change. As the clock tolls, signifying the start of a new day, an internal clock similarly tolls at predictable intervals signifying the time to start anew. Every January, millions get motivated to change. Each spring, they get re-motivated to try again. On birthdays, millions get committed to improve. Each decade of life, they get really committed. There are certain times when people naturally reflect on where they are in life, and it is at these times that they are most receptive to changing the direction they may be going.

All these triggers, though, are knee-jerk reactions to brief stimuli. As a result, the likelihood for long-term change is limited, as the trigger tends to get quickly replaced by other stimuli, prompting the old habits to rear their ugly heads. Acquiring new knowledge about why it is important to change and how this change can be accomplished is the one exception to this rule.

The more you learn the basics of being healthy, the more likely it is that you can change for the long haul. By creating a knowledge base about such health topics as cholesterol, blood pressure, and nutrition, you are building a foundation on which serious change can occur. Most importantly, in order to stay healthy, you need to continually build on this foundation. Just as good investors keep informed about the most recent economic news, healthy people keep informed about medical breakthroughs and general medical trends.

There are many avenues by which you can get accurate health information. You can learn much by reading newspaper articles, health magazines, books, and health letters. You can get a wealth of information from certain websites, television programs, and radio talk shows. You can learn from your own personal experiences, as well as the personal experiences of your family, friends, and co-workers. Then, you can check the relevance of this information to your specific situation by talking with your physician, your de facto private health consultant. The expression *knowledge is power* could never be truer.

The uninformed often feel lost, not even knowing what question they should be asking. As you improve your knowledge about health issues, you are empowering yourself to successfully change, and most importantly, *stay* changed and irreversibly different from the person you were. Developing and maintaining this curiosity about the world of medicine is the first step toward attaining a healthier lifestyle.

Instinctual Drives

When people do start caring and become inspired, it is important that they first try to understand why they behave the way they do. Psychology, the science of human nature, attempts to answer this question. It seems a simple question, yet there are textbooks and textbooks that attempt to answer it. It is a question that has been asked for as long as people have been asking questions. Ironically, in examining the earliest civilizations, their writings and cultures suggest a greater appreciation of the fact that behavior is guided both by intellect and animalistic drives. With its head being that of a man and its body being that of a lion, the Great Sphinx of Egypt highlights this dual nature of the human spirit. The Greek and Roman cultures have similar half-man, half-animal figures that serve to highlight their understanding of the perpetual struggle between human reason and animal passion.

There is a tendency to downplay the animal side of human nature in today's society, especially as it gets more advanced. But, clearly, there are innate urges designed to meet the body's basic needs of survival and immediate pleasure. Although originally designated by Pope Gregory around 600 A.D. as spiritual sins, the seven deadly sins could also serve as an excellent guide to the basic innate animal drives that play such a strong role in human behavior. Pride, envy, anger, greed, sloth, gluttony, and lust represent a good list of things that frequently undermine reason. They are at the root of practically all causes of passion, and they are at the root of most failures to change behaviors. These natural animal drives are shared by everyone to one degree or another. They control the instinctual actions representing behaviors that are not premeditated or preconceived. These forces can be powerfully influential in determining how a person is going to respond in a particular situation. They frequently act as strong currents, invisibly pulling people to act in certain ways. When these forces become irresistible, and ultimately undeniable, they can be referred to as passions.

Through the use of reason, it is hoped that these instinctual drives might be somewhat controlled. Despite being labeled as sins by the church, they are not inherently bad. They are inherently good because they help to ensure survival. It is only when they are excessive in nature, without some active thought to modify them, that they become a problem. If successful behavior change is to occur, it is first important to realize that these natural drives exist, that they are there for the purpose of survival, and that they should not be repressed.

Many people design self-improvement projects that go directly against these natural drives. They starve themselves when they want to lose weight; they exercise themselves to the point of exhaustion when they want to get into shape; and they deny themselves all luxuries when they want some self-restraint in their lives. When these drives are actively suppressed, they only become stronger and stronger until they no longer can be ignored.

Ultimately, both instinctual behavior and reasoned behavior have pleasure as their goal. The difference is that instinctual behavior demands immediate gratification, while reasoned behavior is looking more toward the future. So, the secret to successful, long-term behavior change is to superimpose reason on top of these natural drives, and get them to work synergistically rather than antagonistically.

Categories of Human Behavior

The origins of human behavior can be divided into four categories:

• Reasoned behavior resulting from active thought (i.e., good actions);

• Reasoned behavior resulting from passive thought (i.e., good habits);

• Impulse behavior responding to primal urges (i.e., bad actions);

• Impulse behavior resulting from passive thought (i.e., bad habits).

At the start of a new year, when people are attempting to follow their New Year's resolutions, they are engaging in reasoned behavior that is felt to be in their best interests. As a result, they are consciously trying to act in ways consistent with this goal by performing good actions. The major problem with this type of behavior is that it is difficult to maintain. It is nearly impossible to go through the day thinking about every single behavior or action. The brain gets distracted and the actions fostered by the resolutions gradually stop. On occasion, however, some of these well-intentioned behaviors become part of the routine. When this occurs, people are pursuing reasoned behavior that results from passive thought. They have good habits, even though the original reasons may be long forgotten. As an example, physicians frequently encounter patients in their office who are taking natural supplements, but when pressed, can no longer recall why they started some of them in the first place.

How long it takes for reasoned behavior to become habitual is a matter of debate. Given the right circumstances, most would agree that it takes several weeks for an action to become routine, and the longer the time doing it, the better the chances. Impulse behaviors resulting from the body's innate drives are extremely difficult to ignore. As mentioned previously, it seems that when they are repressed, they only get stronger. Since these behaviors provide immediate gratification, they run the risk of becoming a conditioned response (i.e., a bad habit).

Every day physicians see patients who are predominantly exhibiting impulse behaviors and who have a whole array of bad habits learned through the years. A key point is that most of these people know what constitutes good health habits. They often are well-informed about what they should be doing, and they are well-intentioned. The problem arises because they either don't have a plan or they are unable to execute their plan.

It might be helpful to think in terms of going from point A to point B on a map. These patients know all too well their current health status (point A). They know where they would like it to be (point B). The problem is they just can't get from point A to point B. Either they have no directions (they have no plan), or they don't know how to drive the car (they can't control their bad habits). In essence, then, in order to improve their health, they have to foster the development of good habits, which needs a plan, while also working on identifying and eliminating bad habits.

Develop a Strategy for Success

Once you are committed to improving yourself, you need to develop a strategy to accomplish your goal. Developing a blueprint helps considerably in this mission. While many see this as a mental exercise, if you take the time to write it down, you will be more likely to succeed. Your list should begin by identifying reachable goals, and the reasons why you desired those goals in the first place.

Often, people fail to understand these reasons, and fail to appreciate the true value of what they are trying to attain. The better you understand the why behind your actions, the better your motivation will be when it comes time to perform those actions.

After the goals and reasons have been clearly outlined, you need to construct a time frame. Failure to establish a practical timetable is probably one of the most common stumbling blocks encountered on the road to being healthier. Enthusiasm is often so high that people expect to see results in terms of weeks, rather than months or years. The keys to creating a successful health plan are that you need to keep it simple, work on developing one new habit at a time, and think in terms of months, not weeks.

Eliminate Bad Habits

Often overlooked, the elimination of bad habits is vital to the overall effectiveness of any self-improvement venture. In his book *Leadership*, Mayor Giuliani described how he improved New York City's crime statistics during his tenure as mayor. He spoke of the broken-windows theory at the core of how he approached combating crime while he was in office. His reasoning was, if there is a vacant warehouse on a city street with some broken windows, there is a much higher probability that a citizen, not normally inclined to acting outside the law, will pick up a rock and try to break more windows. He felt that, before the city could improve its numbers with the really bad crimes, such as assault and homicide, it would have to do a better job with the lesser crimes, such as defacing property with graffiti and jumping the turnstiles in the subway. This approach served two purposes. First, it was easier to do—it was a reachable goal. Second, it was readily observable—a sign that change had indeed started to happen.

You can approach any bad habits you may have in much the same way—by focusing on the small infractions. This would serve as a daily reminder that the small actions are really what matter most, and this way you will be much less inclined to stray too far from your health plan. When people are at the end of one of their health crazes, they often give in to all their urges. They become like the person throwing rocks at the building, trying to knock out as many windows as possible.

Teaching an Old Dog . . .

When my wife and I first met, we were highly compatible in nearly all areas, with one notable exception—our taste in sodas. I was a regular soda person, she drank diet soda. In the beginning, when sharing sodas was frowned upon as being a sign of a cheap date, this minor difference flew under the radar, not making much of an impact. But, as we became more serious, and less concerned that we might catch something from each other, we slowly advanced our relationship toward this most intimate of steps.

It started innocently enough while we were waiting in line at the concession stand in the movie theater, when she suggested that we save money, and share our drink. When my wife said "diet," while I voiced "regular" to the cashier, we knew there was a problem. She argued, effectively I might add, that regular soda is loaded with empty calories that lead to unnecessary weight gain. I countered that I can't stand the taste of diet. She promised that after a few days, I wouldn't be able to tell the difference. I wasn't so sure.

Eventually, after many years and many reminders from my wife, I made the change. What ultimately triggered this move was not my reacting to my wife—in reality, people rarely change for the sake of others. No, what caused me to change was my reacting to a number—a number that causes nearly everyone to change.

When my weight registered twenty pounds higher than normal, bells and whistles started ringing in my head signifying the time had definitely come for something to be done. The question at that point became what to do. Instead of going on my usual health kick, during which I am really inspired for a really short time, I decided to do things differently and become really inspired for a really long time by conquering one of my bad habits. So I targeted my soda drinking, and, no surprise, diet soda tasted pretty awful for the first few days, much like the medicine I'd been given as a child.

Most likely the venture would have stopped at this juncture if I hadn't possessed certain knowledge about the calorie content. I knew from reading the label that a 20-ounce regular soda contained about 300 calories. Given that I was drinking at least one, and often two, 20-ounce bottles a day, this was translating to 4,000 calories a week in soda consumption alone. Spurred on by this knowledge, and the fact that the diet soda's taste got better, I continued with my quest.

It took about a week before I couldn't tell the difference between the types of soda. Predictably, my weight dropped, and I learned some valuable lessons about behavior change. First, it's up to the person to change, others can't do it for them. Second, there's always a trigger that causes change to occur. Third, when the trigger does occur, knowing how and why to change will determine ultimate success. Lastly, all things considered, when a wife says it's in her husband's best interests to do something, then it is definitely in his best interests to do something.

Deciding

I last played golf in the summer of 1997, one month before my eldest daughter was born. I had never gotten good at the game, but I did improve enough that I no longer embarrassed myself when I played. I realized, though, that being even a mediocre player would require more time than I could afford to give, so my dad and I decided to play one last game together, my swan song. That round, like most of my rounds of golf, consisted of a wide assortment of good shots, bad shots, missed shots, and lucky shots.

Eventually, after several hours and several lost balls, we found ourselves on the eighteenth tee. My dad, never one to miss a moment, reminded me this would likely be the last hole of golf I would play for quite some time, which, to my ears, sounded more like a reward than a punishment. My opening shot went straight and far, making me wonder aloud how that could have just happened. My next shot, the approach, landed squarely on the green, causing me to literally look around to see if someone else may have hit their ball ahead of us. Two putts later and I finished with a par on the final hole, the perfect ending to a less-than-perfect golf career.

Some could argue this was an ironic ending, with the game taunting me, and tempting me to come back so it could frustrate me some more. I saw it more as poetic, as if the game was giving me something to fondly remember it by until I was able to return to it. The fact that I was able to play well, even for just one hole, suggests I have this ability somewhere deep inside. And with regard to pursuing healthy behaviors, I feel this same ability to succeed exists deep inside everyone. It's within everyone's grasp if they decide to do so. The challenge is to get them to decide.

When I was in high school, I was very impressed with one of my teachers, Mr. Denny, who later went on to become Reverend Denny, a priest. When faced with a decision, he would always say, "Not to decide is to decide." I often think how integral this concept is to human behavior. Everyone is given the opportunity to take active control over their actions, to steer the ship to any destination they want. Some choose to pursue a healthy lifestyle, some choose to pursue an unhealthy one. The problem is that too many people don't make any choice at all.

Tips on Changing Behavior

1. Behavior changes only because something causes it to change. Learn what triggers your behavior to change, and take the first step toward controlling your actions.

2. React, but don't overreact, to your triggers. Change one behavior, not multiple behaviors, at a time, and see the difference this makes.

3. Increase your knowledge base about health topics, and be irreversibly changed from the person you once had been.

4. Your innate drives are there to ensure survival. The more you try to repress them, the stronger they become.

5. Develop a health plan. Keep it simple. Identify one reachable goal. Write out how you will accomplish this goal. And, most important, give yourself a deadline.

6. In line with the broken-windows theory, being disciplined about the small infractions leads to discipline with the large infractions.

7. When faced with a decision, *not deciding is deciding*. Don't let your life be ruled by your innate urges. Decide that you can make a difference.

3

WILLPOWER'S ROLE IN HEALTH

*These are the times that try men's souls. The summer soldier
and sunshine patriot will, in this crisis, shrink from the
service of his country; but he that stands it now
deserves the love and thanks of man.*
—THOMAS PAINE, *THE AMERICAN CRISIS*

I think most of you can recall the summer jobs you once held when
you were younger. They often were thankless and tedious ventures,
but nonetheless they represented so much more. They gave you your
first taste of financial independence and they helped develop a true
appreciation for the time it takes to actually earn a dollar.

In many ways, they symbolized the transition into adulthood. They
offered a challenge to see if you could get the job done, and they highlighted the everlasting spirit of your youth in thinking you could do
just about anything. For many of you, it didn't involve proving anything to yourself, but rather proving something to others. In so doing,
this would stake your claim to early adulthood. It was in this context,
and with much enthusiasm, that I approached a summer job working
with my father.

My dad had his own landscaping business. Each of my brothers had
spent a summer working beside him and then came my turn. Overall,
I really enjoyed those days. It was great to be outside in the sun and
out of the classroom. The feeling of being physically, rather than mentally, tired was refreshing.

One day in particular stands out in my mind. It started as a fairly normal day, with my dad dropping me off at a location to work on a project, while he would go to other sites to get things done. On this day, my project was rather simple, or so it seemed. The delivery truck had inadvertently emptied a load of mulch at the front of a customer's house instead of the back, where it was needed for her impressive flower garden. My task was to move this pile to the back of the house. I had been truly excited to take it on, as it provided an opportunity to get a workout, get some color, and get some listening time with my music, which, at that moment in my life, had started to become a priority. So with a shovel, a wheelbarrow, and a radio, I got started.

The mulch pile, which I can envision to this day, was large but not intimidating, at least not at the start. It was about ten feet across at its base and, at roughly ten feet in height, it was several feet taller than I was. I started out as if I were in a wheelbarrow race at a company picnic. The terrain, a bit rocky, required some maneuvering, but I was quickly able to deliver my first load and practically ran back for a second. I remember wondering what I was going to do to occupy myself until my dad came back after lunch, for it was obvious this project wasn't going to take much time at all. Needless to say, I had underestimated the size and scope of the pile. After about my twentieth trip, my speed slowed considerably, and what was most disheartening was that the pile didn't seem to be shrinking at all. After some trips, it even appeared bigger.

As the morning wore on, it became much hotter. I was definitely no longer running, my shirt was now off, and I began doubting I would ever finish. I had taken a mid-morning break to recoup and restrategize—not that moving a pile of dirt required that much strategy. After the break, I moved somewhat faster, but the big difference was that I had become much more determined. The fun was gone. It became me against the mulch. As the theme song from the movie *Rocky* began echoing in my head, my movements began resembling the slow-motion scenes over which that music is usually played.

After about four hours and well over a hundred wheelbarrow trips, I was a beaten man. The pile had actually been reduced by about half, but mentally it seemed bigger than when I had started. When my dad returned, he had a big smile on his face and laughed when I told him of my legendary battle with the *mountain*—the word *pile* no longer seemed sufficient. After eating lunch, we both attacked the remainder of this mountain. Just having another person to commiserate with did wonders for my psyche, and I was rejuvenated. Together, we finished the job in no time. To this day, I have never had such a feeling of accomplishment as I did when I unloaded that last heap of mulch from the pile into the customer's backyard garden.

Willpower is an interesting concept that is rarely talked about in depth. Failure to achieve goals is frequently blamed on its absence, but otherwise there's not much mention of it in general conversation. Certainly, people are not discussing ways to build up their willpower, for most consider it an inherited quality present from birth. It usually refers to an intangible trait that all people have to one degree or another. It's generally considered to represent a person's level of determination to successfully complete tasks. Although it clearly has a genetic component, it can also be nurtured and strengthened.

My purpose in discussing the story of the pile is to highlight the external factors that influence willpower. The pile can represent any goal you are trying to attain. Its size can represent all that needs to be done to successfully reach that goal. The actual moving of the pile can represent your effort throughout the entire endeavor. For example, the goal of running a marathon might be considered your pile. The size of this pile would then represent all the training, in terms of practice miles that needed to be run, in order to successfully finish the marathon. The effort put forth during this training would be represented by the effort needed to move the pile. Thinking of achieving goals in this manner helps demonstrate all the things that promote willpower and ultimate goal completion.

Building Confidence Equals Building Willpower

Confidence in your ability to achieve a specific goal is probably the most important determiner of your willpower. As long as your confidence remains strong, your willpower remains strong.

Most people approach their self-improvement projects with a great deal of confidence. They strongly believe they will reach their preset goal, and they demonstrate this fact by beginning their project with much enthusiasm and energy. In essence, they start out running with the wheelbarrow. Overflowing with excitement, and laden with high expectations, they can't wait to start seeing results. Unfortunately, though, most things require significant time in order to change. Initial returns are often subtle and very difficult to perceive. It would be similar to returning to a pile that does not appear to be shrinking. It is at this point that doubt might start to appear, and willpower might begin to waver. This failure to see immediate results slows momentum and seriously jeopardizes the likelihood of successful goal attainment.

As is often the case, people significantly underestimate the time and effort needed to meet their stated aims. Basically, when they mentally plan their projects, they create piles that are too big. When people finally come to the realization they are not going to reach their overly ambitious goals, their confidence will have been completely undermined, and their willpower broken.

The time it takes to reach this realization is different for every person. This is where past personal experiences come into play. People tend to repeatedly go after their same goal. They try to move the same pile time and time again. If there is a history of failed attempts, people's confidence gets shaky. It is only natural to expect they will have serious doubts as to whether or not they will ever be able to reach their goal. In subsequent attempts, the time it takes to become aware that a goal will not be met gets shorter and shorter. This may outwardly appear that someone has little or no willpower, when in fact, what they lack is confidence, which is why it is so critical to establish reachable goals in the first place. By creating smaller piles that are easier to move, people are helping to rebuild their confidence.

Confidence can, in many ways, be seen as the subtotal of the mini-victories and mini-failures you experience throughout life. The size of the victory is not as important as the *number* of victories. By accumulating small victories, you can build self-esteem, re-energize willpower, and create momentum for larger victories down the road.

People who are in the habit of making daily lists completely understand this concept of accumulating small victories. Their list is their scorecard. When they cross an item off their list, they have just won a mini-victory. The thrill you can get crossing an item off the list is the same thrill you can get when small goals are achieved—it's the tangible feeling of willpower being re-energized. The important point here is that it doesn't matter if it is a big item or a small item on the list—as long as the item gets crossed off, it gives you the same thrill.

Getting Others to Help Move the Pile

While self-confidence is extremely important, the knowledge that others have confidence in you is an equally powerful motivating tool. This is seen all the time in the world of sports, when, frequently, the less talented team wins the game. Why do these upsets happen so often? The primary reason revolves around the coach's ability to motivate his/her team. During the pre-game speech, the coach attempts to get the team believing that he/she thinks they can win, and believes in them. And the more a team believes this to be the case, the better their chances become.

This phenomenon was showcased on the world stage in 1980, when the United States ice hockey team beat the Soviet Union at the Winter Olympics in Lake Placid. Considered the greatest upset of all time, the United States team defied logic and did the impossible. Their coach, Herb Brooks, had a vision this could be accomplished when no one else did. He constructed a team of players with more determination than talent, and he got them believing. His confidence in them not only enabled them to overachieve, it inspired them to greatness.

The takeaway here is that, by getting others to have confidence in you, you will be significantly bolstering your willpower and improving your chances for ultimate success. You can use the help of others in many different ways. Figuratively speaking, you can enlist other people to help you move your pile. These people may be spouses, family, and/or friends, or they may be someone more professional—trainers, nutritionists, or physicians. Most importantly, the more people that are invited to help, the more likely it is that you that will eventually reach your goal.

Many times people share the same goal. Wanting to exercise, for example, is a common goal shared by many. By exercising with a friend (or a trainer), your long-term adherence to the program will be much better, your enjoyment will be greater, and a joint feeling of accomplishment will be fostered.

Sometimes the assistance may take the form of general interest in what you are trying to accomplish. The knowledge that others care, and that that they will be checking in for progress reports, can be extremely motivating.

Setting a Timeline

Establishing a timetable that includes progress reviews is a very effective way to help you achieve your goal. By definition, this timetable needs to have a starting point, which often proves elusive. You may be extremely knowledgeable about what needs to be done. You may be well-intentioned and well-motivated, but getting started is one of the most difficult aspects of any self-improvement project.

This delay is frequently a result of the tendency to get preoccupied with less important, but more pressing matters. You can get so distracted by the irritating problems of life that you never get to the piles you really want to move, thereby missing the proverbial forest for the trees.

By understanding that the calendar is an effective trigger for initiating behavior change, you can use this knowledge to your advantage. You can plan to have small self-improvement projects begin on Mondays, coinciding with the start of your week. By adopting this approach, you will be considerably increasing your chances of getting started. Similarly, larger projects can be planned for the start of each month; and once a year, on a birthday or another important date, you can schedule general reviews to set up goals for the coming year. Synchronizing behavior change to the calendar can help you transition from being well-intentioned to being well-achieved.

As helpful as it is to have a start date, it is equally beneficial to have a deadline by which to monitor your progress. Too often deadlines get defined in terms of the attainment of specific goals rather than as dates on a calendar. Dieting, for example, is expected to continue until a specific weight loss goal is achieved. For many, this may never happen.

Without a definite time frame, there is loss of focus. It is much more practical for you to reorganize your thinking in such a way that you concentrate on changing specific behaviors during a certain time frame.

The avoidance of late-night snacking over a thirty-day period would be representative of this type of thinking. It establishes a time frame—thirty days—during which the prime focus is on eliminating your bad habit of late-night snacking. At the end of this time frame, you can evaluate if you have been successful. Once you've mastered one behavior, you'll then be able to take on others that would be conducive to achieving your overall goal. Linking the change of a specific behavior to a specific time frame is critical to this process.

Every good businessperson knows that deadlines are needed to improve efficiency. Parkinson's Law highlights this by stating that "work expands to fit the time available for its completion." Make no mistake about it, changing behavior is work. It requires planning, self-training, and lots of effort. Without a definite time frame, it is unlikely that the work needed to be done, would ever get done.

Planning Breaks Helps Move Piles

When people begin their self-improvement projects, their pace is usually that of a sprint. Obviously, the risk of burnout, either mentally or physically, is very high. It is difficult to focus exclusively on something for any prolonged length of time without getting bored and distracted. For this reason, the importance of planning breaks to re-energize cannot be overstated. Whether concentrating on exercising, losing weight, or developing healthy habits, you need to take some days off without feeling guilty. These days are mentally refreshing, and they help to ensure long-term adherence to the plan. Without these planned breaks, the majority of people inevitably end up taking unplanned breaks that run the risk of terminating their effort entirely.

An important concept to bear in mind, though, is that these planned breaks require the discipline of getting back on the program after a break is finished. Rewarding yourself on weekends but reaffirming your commitment on Monday mornings seems to be a good strategy for many people.

Hitting Close to Home

When my second child was born, my mother-in-law, overcome with excitement, passed out in the waiting room outside labor and delivery. Much to her embarrassment, she had to be admitted into the hospital, one floor below her daughter who had just delivered. Everyone in the family felt stressed by this turn of events, but none more so than my wife, who despite being closest in proximity to what was happening, was distant in terms of her ability to help. In an effort to ease the tension she had inadvertently caused, my mother-in-law coaxed a hospital employee to bend the rule that restricted patients from leaving the floor. Her secret rendezvous with her daughter and new grandson was just what was needed to make everyone feel at ease. Ultimately, she recovered, and we were able to laugh at the oddity of having two family members in the hospital at the same time, a feat we hoped never to repeat.

When we were expecting our third child five years later, we thought back to our last hospital experience. "One person in the hospital at a time," we jokingly reminded my mother-in-law. Unfortunately, we didn't think to remind my father as well.

My dad was fairly healthy when he was in his mid-seventies. He had several manageable medical problems, but nothing that really slowed him down. He was still playing golf; in the fall of that same year, he regularly helped in raking leaves; and that winter, he was playing with one of his eight grandchildren every day of the week. No one could have predicted how his underlying health problems would coalesce into the medical version of the perfect storm.

He had, it turned out, three separate but interrelated conditions: emphysema, which usually only affected him during the change of seasons; a blood-vessel condition known as AVM that would occasionally cause his blood vessels to bleed in his small intestine, making him always a little anemic; and aortic stenosis, which meant that the exit door from his heart didn't open as wide as it should have. It was the worsening of his aortic stenosis that started the dominoes falling.

The next winter we noticed a drastic change in my dad. The first sign something was wrong was that he stopped playing with his grandchildren, unusual because he always played with his grandchildren. He looked as though he had gotten older overnight. He walked slower, breathed heavier, and slept longer. He couldn't walk across the room without appearing short of breath. Eventually, he ended up in the hospital, diagnosed with an emphysema flare-up, which would probably have been better described as a general failure to thrive. An ultrasound of his heart done during this hospitalization revealed that his aortic stenosis, which had previously been listed as *moderate,* had progressed beyond severe to the ominous designation of *critical.* Imagine going through a set of automatic sliding doors that only opened wide enough for one person to squeeze through sideways and you will have a good idea what was going on with the valve in my dad's heart. Since it was a mechanical obstruction, no medication would be able to treat this condition and surgery would be the only answer. The problem was, given his emphysema flare-up, he was in no shape for surgery. So, he was discharged home with the hope that, in time, his lungs would slowly improve. But those around him had their doubts.

That spring, my wife heard the words that every woman nine-months pregnant wants to hear: "We're going to induce you, tomorrow." My dad was getting a lung test that same day to see if he had improved any, although it was obvious that he hadn't. When his hemoglobin was found to be 5.0, which was bordering on life-threatening (normal is 12.5), we once again found ourselves in the unenviable position of having two family members in the hospital at the same time, my wife on the fourth floor having our baby, and my dad on the third floor.

My dad's condition, although complex, could be broken down into its basic parts. He needed surgery to fix his valve; that much was clear. His emphysema, made worse by his damaged valve, made the surgery high risk. By bleeding in his small intestine, the blood vessels made the high-risk surgery even riskier. Given that he was getting weaker by the day, waiting for things to improve did not seem to be a good strategy either. In essence, he needed a lot of work done in order to get better. Or, said another way, he had one big pile to move.

If we had focused on the ultimate goal of dad's getting better, it would have been easy to write him off, as he simply had too much wrong with him. Instead, we divided his ultimate goal into smaller, more movable piles. Our first pile was to stabilize him, and we accomplished this by giving him blood, lots of blood, which helped to improve his blood pressure, thereby buying us time to decide what to do next.

Our next pile was the surgery. My dad, who wanted to go down swinging, decided on the surgery. He was transferred to another hospital and put under the care of a surgeon who specialized in high-risk cases. This surgeon immediately commanded the room when he entered, exuding confidence by his body language, speech, and demeanor. He predicted that once the valve was fixed, my dad's breathing and bleeding would both be much better. He set the surgery up for the following week, and asked my mom if she had any questions. Desperate for someone to help her husband, my mom said something to the effect that, "You had me at hello."

The surgery itself went exceedingly well, with no complications. My dad was back in the surgical intensive care unit in no time, and at this point the attention turned toward getting him off the ventilator. This was the pile we feared most, but as luck would have it, this was the pile that was easiest to move. His breathing, as the surgeon had predicted, improved when the valve was fixed. Still, my family, prepared for the worst, was dumbfounded when, only hours after my dad had returned to his room, the doctor proposed removing him from the ventilator and allowing him to breathe on his own. We couldn't believe this turn of events because the surgeon had almost not done the surgery out of fear of this issue, or non-issue as it turned out. It made each of us question other times in our lives when we may have squandered opportunities based on unfounded fears.

Recovering from surgery was the last pile. It was the one that most challenged my dad's willpower, and was the one that proved the most difficult to move. Prior to surgery, all the focus had been on stabilizing my dad, getting him to surgery, and getting him off the ventilator. No one had given much thought to his recovery. As a result, when mentally planning how things were going to go, we had underestimated the work that still needed to be done—we underestimated the size of this pile.

The results of this miscalculation soon became apparent. My dad was hurting so bad from the surgery that he began having doubts he would ever recover, and he relied heavily on others having confidence in him. The doctors, nurses, therapists, even the staff who brought his food trays, all repeated the same theme over and over. "You are doing great. You are going to get better." Their urgings kept him going when it would have been easy for him to quit. His family and friends also helped him get better—they helped him move his pile. And everyone helped in different ways, depending on what talents they had to offer. My mom, never leaving his side, willed him to get better. My brother, knowing how much my dad worried about his wife driving, drove my mom the thirty minutes to and from the hospital every day. Family and friends, unable to be there in person, called daily with words of encouragement. Everyone was figuratively taking a shovel and putting it into dad's pile. They were helping him move it in their own little way. In essence, isn't that what family and friends do? They see each others' piles as their own and they help move them any way they can.

Sensing our initial miscalculation, we then divided his recovery pile into smaller, more movable piles. Short-term goals with well-defined endpoints replaced the long-term goal of recovering from surgery. A timeline was established. Each week, my dad determined to walk farther. At first, he was only able to make it past a few houses on the street, but eventually he was marking his distances in blocks instead of houses. Ultimately, he started feeling better. When the doctor asked how we knew he had turned the corner, we simply answered—he'd started playing with his grandchildren again.

A Lesson in Life

It's funny how life sometimes comes full circle. My dad, fully recovered, was over at my house the other day watching my young son as I was doing some landscaping on my own home. The delivery truck had dumped a load of wood chips at the front of my house instead of the back. (I'm fairly certain they do that on purpose.) Anyway, I found myself in the strange situation of having to move a pile of wood chips with a wheelbarrow, a shovel, and my dad next to me, playing with my son. Having just written the account of my legendary battle with the pile, it was very fresh in my mind, so I decided to ask my dad if he remembered that summer day. He grinned and said, "That was the day I set out to teach you the value of staying in school, Son." He was trying to teach me a life lesson, and obviously it worked because I stayed in school and then some. And even with the rigors of medical school, I still talk about that day as the hardest day of work in my life.

Willpower Tips

1. Make smaller, more movable piles when setting up the goals you want to achieve.

2. Accumulate victories by moving these smaller piles, and watch your confidence grow.

3. Don't forget to enlist others to help. And don't forget to help them where you can.

4. Recognize when people have confidence in you, and get motivated by their words of encouragement.

5. Don't use goal completion as a deadline, for some piles never get completely moved. Rather, set up a definite time frame. If a pile cannot be moved during the time selected, then it should be broken down into smaller parts.

6. Be practical and take planned breaks. Otherwise, unplanned breaks will end the effort.

7. And above all else, don't forget to play with the children, as they will definitely re-energize you.

4

CHOLESTEROL

The Good, the Bad, and the Ugly
—1966 MOVIE STARRING CLINT EASTWOOD

On a daily basis, I do my best Abbott-and-Costello imitation as I attempt to explain what a person's cholesterol numbers really mean. The dialogue usually goes something like this:

"Mr. Smith, your total cholesterol is OK at 190, but we don't really use this number as a guide anymore, so I would just ignore it. Your LDL is your bad cholesterol. Your LDL number is 98. This is good. Therefore, you have good *bad* cholesterol. Your HDL is your good cholesterol. Your number is a low 28. This is bad. So your good cholesterol is bad and your bad cholesterol is good. What does this really mean to you? Well, before I can answer that question, I have to talk to you about your triglyceride level. Your number is 320. This number is a little high. The studies seem to suggest this is bad for you, but they tend to disagree about how bad. Overall, I would have to say that your risk for heart disease is probably high. Mr. Smith . . . Mr. Smith . . ."

Unfortunately, this exchange is closer to reality than satire. I'm fairly certain I have used those exact words on more than one occasion. I question the wisdom of adhering the nicknames good and bad to cholesterol particles whose values can be both good and bad, but it's done universally. It is very easy to see why there is so much confusion, and by extension, frustration, when people attempt to remember and ask, "Which one is my good cholesterol again?"

Why Care about Cholesterol—Learning the Hard Way

Sometimes in life you don't get a second chance. Sometimes, you don't get a mulligan, a do-over, where you can tee up and hit again. And sometimes, you don't even get a warning that trouble may be brewing on the horizon. This was how it was for the best friend of my mom and dad. My uncle, as he was commonly referred to, had always been healthy. He didn't take any medications. He never let anything slow him down, and he certainly had no idea that his life would suddenly end at fifty-four. The doctors said he died of a heart attack, and his family and friends could only say, "But he was so healthy."

Even now, some twenty years later, I still think about my uncle. I often wonder, if he were fifty-four today, would things have somehow turned out differently? There is no doubt that today's medicine, with all its advancements, is much better at postponing death. But the real question is whether or not he would have taken advantage of all these advances.

When people are feeling well, it is extremely difficult to convince them they should make changes. While a good philosophy in many life situations, the "don't fix it if it's not broken" mentality is more like denial in medical situations, and it's a hard one to break. In these circumstances, people have to be shown how they are *at high risk* for developing a problem before they will likely take any action. Defining this risk is the critical step in the process. Those identified as possibly being in danger will likely seek ways to improve their situation; those not so identified, who don't listen to their bodies, will not know they should change their ways. For people who need outside help to figure out what is going on with their bodies, doctors are getting better and better at identifying those at risk. They have many tools at their disposal to help with the process, but the one they always use first is the cholesterol test.

Cholesterol—What Is It Good For?

Cholesterol is a substance needed by the body to perform several functions. Its use in the development of cell membranes is arguably its most important job. The cell is the building block of life. Assisting in its construction is a role that cannot be underestimated. Cholesterol is also vital to the creation of estrogen, testosterone, and other hormones. It is produced by the liver in the human body, but it is also ingested in any food that is a byproduct of animals. It began being routinely screened as a laboratory test in the 1970s. Cholesterol has always been measured *by weight,* and the accepted standard of reporting the result came to be *milligrams* (of cholesterol) per *1 deciliter* (of blood).

It soon became readily apparent that cholesterol did not mix well with blood. Therefore, it had to be transported in some type of vehicle, or carrier molecule. With the discovery of this molecule, the term *lipoprotein* was born. Lipoprotein is simply the conjoining of two substances—lipids (i.e., cholesterol) plus the carrier protein molecule. This protein functions as a taxicab taking the cholesterol around the body.

As more studies were done, it became obvious there was more than one type of carrier protein—in fact, they found five. Therefore, starting in the early 1980s, the terms *HDL* and *LDL* began to be used. They subdivided the lipoproteins by their relative densities, leading to the less-than-imaginative names high-density lipoprotein (HDL), low-density lipoprotein (LDL), intermediate-density lipoprotein (IDL), very-low-density lipoprotein (VLDL), and chylomicrons.

Laboratories still report each of these subclasses by weight in order to quantify how much of each subclass is available. HDL, the good cholesterol subclass, is responsible for helping to remove the cholesterol from your body. The bigger your army of HDL, the better your chances are of keeping your arteries clean.

The rest of the lipoproteins are considered atherogenic, or capable of promoting plaque development. LDL, the bad cholesterol, is primarily responsible for the transportation of cholesterol to the artery wall. It is the LDL level that has come to be the standard by which your cholesterol numbers are judged.

Size Matters

Newer technology is able to subdivide these lipoprotein classes even further. It is possible to base these subdivisions on the *actual number* of individual particles and on *the size* of each particle.[1] The blood test that measures the numbers of particles is called a nuclear magnetic resonance (NMR) test, and the test that measures the size of particles is known as a vertical auto profile (VAP) analysis.

These further distinctions have significant potential implications with regard to how likely you may be to develop heart disease. The smaller the particles, the more likely it is that you will form plaque in your arteries. This is because the smaller particles are better able to penetrate beneath the surface of the artery. Imagine, if you will, that the inside of your artery is similar to a painted wall. The cholesterol particles do not stick to the paint, but rather slip through the cracks, reaching the inner wall. This then triggers the inflammatory cascade, with resultant plaque formation, or bubbling in the paint.

Another way to think about this concept is to appreciate the fact that one person's LDL level of 130 may be vastly different from another person's LDL level of 130. One person may have an increased number of smaller LDL particles, while the other person may have fewer, but bigger, particles. In laboratory terms, the net result is that both collections of LDL particles equal a weight of 130 milligrams. In practical terms (assuming everything else about the two people is equal), the net result is that the person with smaller particles will be much more likely to develop plaque and heart disease. This same fractionation can be done to the HDL particles, thereby conferring a different risk based on their size and number. This means one person's HDL of 50 may be vastly different from another person's HDL of 50. The first person may have primarily large-sized HDL particles, which are more protective and effective at keeping his or her arteries clean, while the second person may have smaller-sized HDL particles, making him or her more vulnerable to forming plaque. In the second scenario, the high total HDL is deceptive, and can fool someone into thinking they are being protected, when they really are not.

Cholesterol—What Is It Bad For?

Atherosclerosis refers to the development of plaque in the blood vessels (i.e., arteries). It can occur in any artery, and it frequently occurs in multiple arteries in different locations of the body. As is the case for every organ, the heart needs a continuous supply of blood, and by extension, oxygen in order to keep working. Any plaque that develops in the arteries feeding the heart causes a blockage of this continuous flow. Many people think plaque is formed by an accumulation of cholesterol sticking to the inside wall of an artery. This is not really what happens. Think of the inside of the artery as a brick-lined tunnel, with the bricks representing the cells that make up the lining of the artery. Cholesterol does not actually stick to this brick wall of the artery, but rather delves *underneath* the damaged brick-wall surface, or between or through the damaged brick wall's surface cells.[2]

A number of conditions can damage these surface-lining cells. The major players are generally thought to include high blood pressure, smoking, diabetes, infections, and even cholesterol molecules, such as LDL and LPa (another undesirable low-density lipoprotein), themselves. When the cholesterol component breaks through the surface cells and gets into the lining of the artery, a cascading inflammatory reaction results. This phenomenon can be identified in the laboratory by measuring C-reactive protein (CRP) levels, with the higher levels corresponding to higher plaque burdens. The end result of this cascade of inflammatory reactions is the formation of plaque, bulging both inward and outward from the wall of the artery.

In many ways, the inflammatory cascade can be considered every bit as bad as the cholesterol molecule that may have triggered the cascade in the first place. Said another way, cholesterol is the spark that may or may not ignite the inflammatory process. In some cases, the spark catches; in others it doesn't. This might help explain why one person with a cholesterol reading in the range of 225 milligrams goes on to have recurrent heart attacks, while another person, whose cholesterol is in the same range, does not. In the first case, the spark ignited the inflammatory process. In the second case, it didn't.

Another common misconception is thinking that a 75 percent blockage in an artery is always worse to have than a 30 percent blockage. This is not necessarily the case. A 75 percent blockage tends to be a stable plaque, unlikely to rupture or get torn away from the wall of the artery. It usually does not restrict blood flow while a person is at rest and the heart is beating slowly. With exercise, though, the 75 percent blockage would likely begin obstructing flow, and causing problems. When this happens, an area of heart muscle would not get the blood flow it needs. Chest pain, referred to as angina, would predictably follow, causing the person to stop what they were doing, and seek medical attention. Therefore, in this case, angina is beneficial in that it gives a warning that trouble may be on the way.

The 30 percent blockage, on the other hand, would not cause angina because it would not obstruct any blood flow, even with vigorous exercise. Without the benefit of angina, there'd be no warning that plaque may be accumulating in the heart's arteries. The problem arises in the fact that the 30 percent lesion may be an immature plaque with the potential to suddenly rupture. With no previous symptoms, it can go from 30 to 100 percent blocked in seconds. This would be represented by the seemingly healthy, active male who suddenly drops dead of a heart attack while mowing the lawn. This man could have gone to a cardiologist the day before he collapsed; he could have successfully passed a stress test; and he could have been able to run a marathon. And yet, despite all these positive indicators, he would still have dropped dead from a heart attack.

The stress test is only designed to detect significant blockages (usually 70 percent or greater). By definition, stress tests would not find the lesser plaques, and, often, a normal stress test can give a false sense of security. In order to take proper corrective measures, it is important to understand you still may be at risk. If your cholesterol readings are not as good as they might be, you need to take them seriously and appreciate the value in attempting to improve their level.

1984—Becoming Public Health Enemy Number One

When did cholesterol start getting a bad reputation? It had been suspected of being a major player in the development of plaque for quite some time, but this was not scientifically proven until the 1980s. In January 1984, the landmark Lipid Research Clinics Coronary Primary Prevention Trial showed that lowering high cholesterol reduced the risk of getting heart disease.[3]

After that, in 1985, the National Institutes of Health (NIH) created the National Cholesterol Education Program (NCEP) whose primary mission was, and still is, to educate both physicians and their patients regarding cholesterol management based on the latest scientific evidence. By all accounts, the NCEP would have to be considered incredibly successful. Since its inception, its recommendations have been the standard of care with regards to lipid management. More impressively, statistics from the 1980s and 1990s have demonstrated both a decrease in total cholesterol numbers for the country as a whole, and a decrease in the death rate from heart disease in particular.

The initial 1984 Lipid Research Clinics Coronary Primary Prevention Trial has been followed by mountains of good, objective studies evaluating many different aspects of the cholesterol issue. It would be impossible to name them all, but it may be helpful to mention a few of the major ones in order for you to gain confidence in the recommendations you may be hearing from your doctor. (Caveat here before I start: Cholesterol studies rival the federal government in their excessive use of acronyms to cleverly name themselves.)

In the mid-1990s, a series of major studies arrived that addressed both primary prevention (before known heart problems) and secondary prevention (after known heart problems) in people with varying degrees of high cholesterol. Some particularly important studies include the West of Scotland Coronary Prevention Study (WOSCOPS), the Cholesterol and Recurrent Events Trial (CARE), the Long-Term Intervention with Pravastatin in Ischemic Disease (LIPID), and the Scandinavian Simvastatin Survival Study (4S).[4,5,6,7]

These studies conclusively demonstrated marked reductions in heart problems, both new and recurrent, when cholesterol had been intentionally lowered with medications.[8]

This benefit from the use of medications was shown time and again. These respected studies are still quoted by experts today because of their objectivity, the quality of their design, and their patient sample size. Most physicians, after reviewing these studies, have no doubt that the benefit of lowering cholesterol has been proved.

Obviously not all studies are created equal. There have been thousands of research projects looking at the cholesterol question. Some have been poorly designed. Some did not involve a large sample size. Many have an inherent bias resulting from being sponsored by a drug company, which spent millions on the design, development, and research of a particular medication. As a result, how can you determine the best course of action to follow?

This is where the National Cholesterol Education Program (NCEP) has an important role. Functioning as an arm of the National Institutes of Health (NIH), the NCEP basically represents a group of leading experts who are continually reviewing the studies being reported. In many ways, these experts serve as consultants for physicians on the front lines, and by extension, as consultants for the patients these physicians serve. They weed through the mountains of new studies looking for quality of study design, reproducibility of results, and potential relevance to clinical practice. When enough new evidence surfaces to conclusively demonstrate that a change in cholesterol management is required, the NCEP issues new treatment recommendations under the heading of Adult Treatment Panel (ATP).

On many laboratory reports, these treatment guidelines are printed underneath the cholesterol numbers. To date, there have been three issuances of these guidelines, ATP I, ATP II, and ATP III. The first guidelines, ATP I, were issued around the time that the NCEP was created in the late 1980s; ATP II guidelines were reported in 1993; ATP III guidelines, the current standard, were initially set forth in May 2001, and later revised, by way of an addendum, in April 2004.

Cholesterol Management—A Risky Business

From its inception, the NCEP has relied on a physician's ability to estimate an individual's risk of ultimately developing heart disease—the cholesterol goals, as set forth by the commission, are, in fact, heavily contingent on this assessment. Ideally, those most in danger will be identified, and will, as a result, be appropriately treated. Often, however, this is easier said than done.

Much of the confusion surrounding the cholesterol issue results from this imperfect process of risk stratification. The blood levels of LDL, HDL, and triglycerides, the ratio of LDL over HDL, the history of smoking, the existence of other medical conditions such as diabetes and hypertension, and the presence of heart disease in other family members are just some of the data used by the physician to approximate this risk.

Over the years, it has become apparent that some indicators are better predictors than others. As more time and money are invested in improving this process, physicians will be better able to identify those most in need of treatment, and of what sort. Practically speaking, treatment decisions tend to be based solely on your total cholesterol number, rather than on your overall risk of having a heart attack. This is a mistake as it oversimplifies a complex process. As a result, many people are treated unnecessarily when their risk is quite low, while others are falsely reassured that everything is OK when their risk might be quite high. Your energies should be focused on learning your risk so you can take the appropriate measures to reduce it. The key is accurately determining your risk.

To better understand risk stratification, it may be helpful to look at how the car insurance agents determine premiums. Their business is literally dependent on identifying those drivers most at risk of having an accident. In order to do this successfully, they must be able to analyze multiple variables simultaneously, understanding that each, in their own little way, contributes to someone's overall risk.

Age, sex, and overall driving experience are just some of the things taken into consideration when calculating risk. From reviewing this data, the likelihood of accidents can be accurately predicted. The same can be done for predicting heart attacks. Someone with a high level of bad cholesterol in their blood would be equal to the person known to drive fast on the highway. Each would be at a higher risk of having an accident. If the person also had diabetes, then it would be equal to the fast driver known to change lanes frequently. The risk would be that much higher. Add high blood pressure to the mix, and the driver would be talking on a cellphone. Add smoking, and the driver just dropped his cell phone, and was looking to pick it up. In each case, it is easy to appreciate that over a period of time, the risk of car accidents or heart attacks becomes increasingly more likely as more variables are added to the list.

The key point, though, is the time frame. It would be impossible to predict someone having a car accident or a heart attack within the next couple of months, no matter how poor the indicators. In both these instances, risk would be better defined in years, rather than months. This delay in seeing adverse results has its pros and cons. On the one hand, it affords plenty of time during which changes can be made to avoid disaster. But, on the other hand, it affords plenty of time during which a person can become complacent. Convincing people they should act now rather than later is the real challenge doctors face with the cholesterol issue.

LDL Cholesterol—How Low Should It Go?

The ATP I, ATP II, and ATP III guidelines all use LDL levels as the primary goal of therapy. The major studies have consistently shown that lowering LDL cholesterol, usually with medications, reduces mortality, heart attacks, and strokes, making it an obvious choice on which to base recommendations. ATP III, the current standard, distinguishes itself from its predecessors by emphasizing primary prevention, that is, prevention of the first heart attack. It classifies an LDL level less than 100 as optimal, and in its addendum in April 2004, it listed an LDL goal of less than 70 as a *reasonable* treatment strategy in those who are at high risk for recurrent heart disease.[9]

Anyone who has ever had a heart attack, undergone angioplasty, or has a history of diabetes, aneurysms, or other circulatory problems should do everything possible to get her or his LDL cholesterol at least below 100. This is an absolute must.

A new addition to the ATP-III guidelines is the inclusion of the ten-year risk assessment with the Framingham scoring system. This scoring system is derived from the Framingham Heart Study, which followed thousands of men and women over their lifetimes, recording their demographic data and noting whether they had ever had a heart attack. This information enabled physicians to estimate the risk of any individual who might share characteristics similar to those in the original study. Simply by inputting certain vital statistics, such as age, sex, and smoking history, physicians are able to calculate a person's ten-year risk for developing heart disease. A value greater than 20 percent is considered very high, and it is recommended that these people also lower their LDL number to at least below 100, usually with the help of medications.

ATP III defines an LDL level of less than 130 as *near* optimal. If a person has two or more established risk factors, then it is imperative to get the LDL below 130 (with medication if necessary). The major risk factors, as outlined in the ATP III report, include:

1. Cigarette smoking;

2. Blood pressure above 140/90 mm Hg or on blood-pressure medication;

3. Low HDL less than 40;

4. Early family history of heart disease;

5. Age greater than forty-five years for men and fifty-five for women.

Generally, anyone with a ten-year Framingham score that predicts a 10 to 20 percent risk of developing heart disease within the next ten years would also have an LDL less than 130 as their goal.

Finally, ATP III defines an LDL level between 130 and 159 as borderline high. If a person is felt to have a low risk for developing heart disease, which would correspond to a Framingham score projecting to a less than 10 percent risk over the next ten years, then it is advisable to keep the LDL below 160.

Therefore, the recommended LDL goal is clearly dependent on risk assessment. Simply, high risk or established heart disease mandates an LDL at least below 100; moderate risk changes the goal to less than 130; and low risk tolerates a goal less than 160.

A Little TLC

How can you reach these goals? As an initial approach, physicians have always advocated diet, weight loss, and exercise. Unfortunately, these recommendations depend on a change of habits which, as mentioned earlier, is very difficult to do. Many physicians have abandoned even starting with the diet-and-exercise approach. They see it as a waste of time, and feel it unlikely that any significant gains can be made by recommending it. The NCEP, recognizing the stigma associated with the term diet and exercise, uses the more socially acceptable *therapeutic lifestyle changes* (TLC) when describing the non-medical approach to improving a person's numbers. ATP III recommends a TLC diet that includes a reduction of saturated fats to less than 7 percent of total calories, a reduction in cholesterol intake to less than 200 milligrams per day, an increase in plant sterols to 2 grams a day, and an increase in soluble fiber to 10–25 grams a day. Generally, it is felt that if significant progress with the TLC program is not made within three months, then consideration should be made for drug therapy to get the person to his or her allotted goal.

Despite doing everything as directed, many people can still have high cholesterol numbers. The primary driving force behind cholesterol levels tends to be genetics. Approximately 70 percent of the cholesterol the body uses is derived from its production by the liver. Only 30 percent actually comes from the diet. Therefore, you could conceivably eat everything right, exercise regularly, and have a normal weight, yet still have high numbers. This helps to explain the fact that cholesterol medication tends to be for the long-term as people cannot change their genes.

Medications—Preventing the Heart from Attacking

There are several types of cholesterol medications, but the statin class would be considered the real kingpin in terms of its potency and its effectiveness. The first statin appeared on the market in the late 1980s. It was soon followed by five new statin drugs in the 1990s. They work by inhibiting the production of cholesterol by the liver. Given that there is less cholesterol inside itself, the liver places more LDL receptors on its surface, which help to remove LDL cholesterol from the bloodstream. It was originally thought that all the benefit derived from statins was from this LDL-lowering effect, which, in essence, helped to eliminate the spark that ignites plaque formation.

Emerging data, however, seems to suggest the statins may have some behind-the-scenes effects that may not be fully represented by the degree to which they lower LDL cholesterol. It appears they somehow seem to stabilize plaque that had already been formed, making a sudden rupture of plaque much less likely.[10]

The statins also appear to blunt the inflammatory reaction that plays such a big role in the formation of plaque in the first place. Some of the statins have demonstrated this phenomenon by showing reductions in C-reactive protein (CRP), a molecule thought to be highly involved in this inflammatory process. Essentially, the statins help prevent new plaque from forming and old plaque from causing damage. This translates into marked reductions in both heart attacks and strokes.

Boldly Going Where No Man Has Gone Before

Emerging new technology may radically change the approach to cholesterol management. Risk stratification is a complex process looking at multiple variables. Ultimately, though, after all the analysis is complete, the estimation of risk is just what the name implies—an estimation. It may be an educated guess, but it is still a guess nonetheless. Previously, the only way to know for sure if any plaque had formed on arteries was to perform a heart catherization, an invasive procedure that most people want to avoid.

Then, in 1999, the Food and Drug Administration (FDA) approved electron-beam computed tomography (EBCT), a non-invasive way to see if there is any plaque forming around the heart arteries. Think of this technology as a new and improved computed tomography (CT) scan that literally takes only a few minutes to perform and interpret.

In an EBCT scan, calcium lights up as white and frequently lines plaque. Therefore, if there is significant plaque buildup, there will be an elevated calcium score. The higher the calcium score, the more plaque likely to be present. There are some limitations to the test. After all is said and done, it, too, is just an estimation or approximation of plaque, but it does appear to give a more accurate estimation than other tools used for this purpose.

There are different types of EBCT scans offering varying degrees of resolution. The first scans were all of the 16-slice variety. These would be similar to the images you would see if you used a 2-pixel digital camera. They offer pictures of fair quality, giving a rough approximation of what may be happening inside your arteries.

Then there is the 64-slice scan. This gives an incredible picture, and would be similar to moving up to a 6-pixel digital camera. When an IV contrast agent is added, this scan can provide a fairly good estimate of overall plaque burden, and more impressively, it can show specific areas of blockage in the arteries, even going so far as to report the percentage of narrowing.

There is still controversy in the medical community regarding how to use this impressive technology. Some argue that these scans are a waste of your money because they don't change what you ultimately are going to do. Others believe these scans could change your level of aggressiveness, making you more likely to stay with your diet, more determined to keep with your exercise program, or more willing to explore other treatment options.

As a general rule, it is always a good idea to ask yourself what you are going to do with the result of any test before having it done. This is especially true when thinking about doing a scan of your heart. That being said, there are times when the test is very useful, and may alter what you do. In these situations, you need to know that the test exists, and should at least consider having it done.

For starters, when calculating your ten-year risk of having a heart attack, if your risk is found to be intermediate, that is, between 10 and 20 percent, then you may want to do the test. The rationale is that high-risk individuals, people whose risk is greater than 20 percent, should already be doing everything in their power to lower the risk. Therefore, the test wouldn't add anything, and shouldn't be done. For low-risk individuals, those with a ten-year risk of less than 10 percent, the test is unlikely to change anything and shouldn't be done. Why expose yourself to unnecessary radiation if your chances of having a problem are so low? But, it is the people in the intermediate-risk group who have the most to benefit, as they may be able to adopt a more aggressive stance regarding modifying their risk factors.

Another group who might benefit would be those with a strong family history of early heart disease. If your brother, sister, mother, or father had a heart attack at a young age, then your genetics may be working against you, and the scan will alert you earlier that you may need to take some precautions.

Lastly, if your doctor is concerned about your cholesterol numbers and is insisting that you take medication, but you are reluctant, the test may help strengthen your argument that you could continue with dietary measures.

In years past, physicians have been reluctant to commit people to long-term medication when their numbers weren't that high. With the EBCT, there is another option. The test can be performed to see if there is any significant elevation in the calcium score. If there is a strong indicator suggesting the existence of plaque, any plaque, it becomes much easier to start a medication and feel comfortable with the choice. In any case, the EBCT result may prove to be a vital piece of information in the decision process, swinging people toward or away from a certain therapy.

When Is There a Heart Problem?

Recently, I saw a patient in the office who frequently voiced her strong aversion to medications. Unfortunately, she had a strong family history of heart disease, and she also had an LDL level greater than 200 milligrams, which is very high. When her numbers did not substantially improve with diet and exercise, I sent her for a CT scan of her heart's arteries in an effort to convince her that medication was warranted in her case. She scored poorly—90 percent of women her age had a better score than hers. After being informed of this, she still expressed a desire to avoid medication, so she was sent to a cardiologist to get a specialist's opinion. I spoke with her after her appointment. She didn't particularly like the cardiologist because he talked to her as if she "had a heart problem." What I find most interesting about that statement is that it involves the bigger question: When does someone have a heart problem? Nearly everyone thinks their heart condition starts the day they are taken into the emergency room with chest pain. I would argue that their heart problem started ten to fifteen years earlier when the plaque had just started forming. In my patient's case, she reluctantly consented to taking medication, eventually coming to the conclusion this was the right thing for her to do.

One Step Forward, Two Steps Back?

It was November a few years ago and the Colts were playing the Patriots on Monday Night Football. All seemed right in the world. Then the phone rang. My Uncle B, who had been well, was being rushed to the hospital. He had had a heart attack and he died that same night at only sixty-five years of age. It would seem, despite all our advancements, that we still have a long way to go.

Cholesterol Tips

1. Get your cholesterol checked, and if it is abnormal, get it checked regularly.

2. Avoid using the very common terms good cholesterol and bad cholesterol, as they can be confusing. Think in terms of HDL and LDL instead. The HDL should be *high*, the LDL should be *low*.

3. Size matters. The bigger the HDL and LDL particles, the better it is; the smaller the particles, the worse it is. If you are at higher risk for developing heart disease, and are not taking any medication, ask your doctor about possibly getting the VAP blood test to measure the size of your particles.

4. With your doctor's help, calculate your ten-year risk of having a heart attack. If it is greater than 20 percent, you should be on medication.

5. If you have a strong family history of heart disease, and your cholesterol numbers are not that bad, talk to your doctor about possibly getting some EBCT imaging of your heart's arteries.

6. Practice a little TLC (therapeutic lifestyle change). Diet and watch your pharmacy bill slim down; exercise and watch your heart beat more soundly. By following the American Heart Association's recommendations for diet and exercise, you'll be much less likely to have a heart attack.

7. Time is on your side, so take advantage of it. Plaque doesn't develop overnight, but rather it develops over years. The difference between opportunity and missed opportunity may well be found in whether you check your cholesterol or not.

I dedicate this chapter in memory of Edward McGinley (Uncle Eddie), 1930–1984, and William Carlin (Uncle B), 1940–2005

5

EXERCISE

Pay yourself first.
—David Chilton, *The Wealthy Barber*

Every vacation I hope to start an exercise routine and get back in shape. I make "the pledge" as my wife mockingly refers to it. It usually goes something like, "I'm going to wake up early to run this year." I have to use the modifier "this year" because, as the phrase implies, I have failed to wake up early during previous vacations. In fact, despite good intentions, I have never been good at waking up early to exercise; the power of the bed is just too strong. This past year, I was determined that things would be different. I was determined not to be awakened by my wife again asking how my imaginary run had been. This was the year that things were going to change, or so I told myself. When my alarm rang, I crawled out of bed, dressed in the hall-way, cursed several times, and eventually began the slow jog down the street. It was a beautiful summer day, I was down at the Jersey shore, and decided to run along the beach. I joined the throng of early morning exercisers, feeling guilty, as if I were intruding in their elite club. After about two miles, I had to stop because I couldn't go any farther. All right, it was probably closer to one mile. When I finally made it back home (I had to walk halfway back), I felt like a person who hadn't run in some time. I was winded, soaked in sweat, and unable to talk. My sister-in-law, who happened to see me as I walked in the door, said I looked like the person from the movie *Beaches*—the extremely pale woman dying from heart failure, who couldn't walk across the room without appearing short of breath. I didn't know if I should be more offended by the remark or more embarrassed by being a man who happened to watch that movie. Despite my initial poor showing, I continued to jog every day during the rest of my vacation.

From just this brief period of sustained exercise, I was able to draw several conclusions. First, I was able to go a little farther, a little faster, a little easier, with each jogging session. This ability to do more with continued training has always amazed me about exercise. Second, the primary short-term reward was how good it made me feel. It lifted my mood, increased my energy level, and boosted my self-esteem. It was incredible how twenty minutes of exercise in the morning could still pay dividends, eight to twelve hours later in the day. Finally, although often overlooked, exercise has the strong effect of promoting me (along with others) to choose additional healthy behaviors. I found myself much more inclined to make better choices regarding the foods I ate. The french fries, burgers, and donuts were not nearly as appealing after sweating earlier in the day. I was much more likely to allocate more time for sleep because I was more physically fatigued from my work-out. Equally important, the quality of my sleep improved because my body went into a deeper, more refreshing sleep. Lastly, once my body was primed with exercise, I was more likely to pursue other physical activities.

Overall, I actively thought about being healthier, and my actions changed accordingly. The real challenge for me was finding the time to incorporate exercise into the non-vacation world that encompassed the other fifty weeks of the year. Studies show I am not alone in that.

Drinking from the Fountain of Youth

One of my oldest patients, both in terms of his age and the time he has been seeing me, came into the office complaining of being tired. Normally, he never complained, which made his symptoms all the more concerning. He said that his gait was slower; his stamina was down; and he was feeling generally weak. A friend had told him he was finally looking his age, which at ninety-four, he hadn't found too complimentary, prompting him to make his appointment.

He couldn't point to any one thing that may have triggered his decline. Instead, he said he had noted a gradual onset of the symptoms over the preceding several months. Fortunately, his exam was normal, including routine blood work that had been ordered prior to his visit. Upon further questioning, it was found that inclement weather during the winter had disrupted his regular routine of walking each morning, a habit he said he had been unable to restart. It soon became obvious that his tiredness was likely the result of his recent inactivity. Therefore, the treatment, believe it or not, was to send this ninety-four-year-old man to the gym, which was exactly what I did.

With a doctor's note in hand, my patient proudly marched into the fitness center to begin his closely supervised exercise routine. Nike's "Just Do It" slogan would never be better epitomized. He was embraced warmly by the gym's staff, and he excelled in the program they designed for him. By six weeks, his tiredness had completely abated, and he felt well enough to resume golfing, a sport he has always loved. By exercising, he was keeping himself young and able to do all that he wanted.

Let's Get Physical—Thirty Minutes a Day, Every Day

It is estimated that only 20 percent of Americans are achieving their recommended daily allotment of physical activity. This is in spite of major efforts put forth by the public health agencies to promote education and increase awareness about its benefits. As the National Institutes of Health (NIH) has set the gold standard for the proper management of cholesterol, the Centers for Disease Control and Prevention (CDC) and the American College of Sports Medicine (ACSM) have jointly set the standards for physical activity levels.

In February 1995, a committee of twenty experts selected by the CDC and the ACSM came together and issued a public health message that is still in effect today. They concluded that "every U.S. adult should accumulate thirty minutes or more of moderate-intensity physical activity on most, preferably all, days of the week."[1]

The wording of this statement is notable by the absence of the word exercise. People do not have to go to the gym, hire a personal trainer, or even change into exercise clothes to start meeting their recommended daily allotment. Physical activity is defined as "any bodily movements produced by skeletal muscles that result in energy (calorie) expenditure."[2]

Moderate-intensity physical activity would be equal to brisk walking at three to four miles per hour. This would be equal to a pace slightly faster than a stroll, during which leisurely conversation gets difficult. A major addition to the recommendation is the word *accumulate.* It is not necessary to perform any activity for a thirty-minute continuous session. Instead, you can achieve your goal by gradually collecting minutes over the course of your average day. Therefore, small decisions, such as parking farther from the store, always using the steps, and taking a ten-minute power walk at lunch can start really adding up. By reaching your daily thirty-minute goal, you can start to reap some very important health benefits, such as lowering the incidence of first heart attacks, lowering the incidence of death from recurrent heart attacks, and lowering your chances of dying from any cause.[3,4,5,6]

As the total amount of physical activity increases, either by higher intensity workouts or by acquiring more minutes of lesser intensity activity, the potential benefits also increase. What should not be overlooked, though, is that those who have the most to gain from increasing their activity are those who are the most sedentary.[7]

For example, the net health benefit would be much greater for the previously inactive person who starts walking, than for the regular jogger who increases the distance of his/her run from three to five miles a day.

What Derails Many Exercise Programs?

Before discussing specifics about the benefits of exercise, it is important to understand that many people start exercising with false expectations of what their exercising might bring. The vast majority expect and want to lose weight quickly, and, as a result, they pursue an overly aggressive program of vigorous exercise, three to four days a week.

In many ways, they may be thought of as a train speeding down a track. The question is whether they are heading for the right destination. It is easy to imagine the brakes of that train beginning to screech as the weight fails to come down. They console themselves by remembering the adage, muscle weighs more than fat, and they figure that must be the reason for the lack of immediate results. Frequently, after only a month of regular high-intensity workouts, the train gets derailed and the exercise program stops. What causes this sudden stoppage? The actual weight goes up a few pounds, they get completely discouraged, their egos get deflated, and their motivation gets lost. The reason for their failure was that the train was heading toward the wrong station. By itself, without diet and other lifestyle changes, exercise is not effective as a quick weight-loss tool.

It is helpful to think of weight management in terms of calories or energy units. In order to lose one pound of weight, you have to burn 3,500 calories. A fairly vigorous workout for thirty to forty-five minutes would likely consume only 350 calories. Assuming that your diet is unchanged, you would have to perform this vigorous workout for ten days in a row in order to lose one pound of weight.

Often when people start an exercise program, they also simultaneously change their diet. Any weight loss that might follow would much more likely be from the change in diet rather than the increased exercise. Although not a short-term answer, exercise can, however, be very helpful for successful long-term weight management.[8]

This has been demonstrated time and again, particularly by an analysis of participants in the National Weight Control Registry (NWCR), a database established in 1994. In order to be eligible, its members must maintain a thirty-pound weight loss, at least. More than 90 percent of the registry's participants reported that they depended on increased physical activity to maintain their weight loss over time.

It should be noted, though, that on average, they reported devoting more than an hour a day to moderate-intensity workouts, or at least double the recommended amount. If you begin an exercise program with an unrealistic expectation, such as rapid weight loss, then it is likely you will stop the program as soon as you perceive your goals are not being met.

More Exercise, Less Medication

The health benefits of regular exercise are immeasurable. In addition to the aforementioned decrease in heart disease and death, exercise improves blood pressure and decreases the chances of getting diabetes. Studies have shown a greater than seven-point drop in blood pressure readings and a more than 50 percent reduction in the development of diabetes in individuals who were physically active.[9,10]

Studies have also shown improvements in depression, improvements in osteoporosis, and the possible reductions of certain cancers, such as cancers of the breast and colon.[11,12,13,14]

By pursuing a physically active lifestyle, you can significantly reduce your chance of needing medications to treat these medical conditions. This decision to take control of your life can translate into less medication, less side effects from medication, less money spent on health insurance premiums, less restriction of activities, and yes, less time being dead.

Excuses, Excuses, Excuses . . .

Given all the potential benefits, why do only one in five Americans reach the minimum recommended level of physical activity? Surprisingly, awareness of benefits does not seem to have much impact on whether anyone engages in regular exercise.[15]

Most people are aware that exercise is good for them. Most people intend to exercise. Most people don't exercise. Some argue that it's just too inconvenient. The large stockpile of unused workout equipment in many homes would argue against this claim. Is it strictly a matter of lack of time? This is the number-one reason cited for not exercising, and there is some validity to this statement.

Despite living in this time period, with all its advances and time-saving technologies, people seem to have less rather than more free time to pursue recreational activity. They are leaving for work earlier, arriving home from work later, and frequently extending their working hours into the weekend. As a result, there doesn't seem to be much time or energy remaining to pursue a regular fitness program. All too often, though, this lack of time is conveniently used as an excuse for never having developed good habits. This may be demonstrated by studying the retired and semi-retired who have all the time in the world. Their exercise pattern and physical activity levels tend to be exactly the same as they had been when time was scarce.

For working-age people, when free time does suddenly become available, they don't usually start exercising. It is not lack of time, it is not that people are unaware of its value, it is not a matter of inconvenience. What it comes right down to is that people don't exercise because *they haven't developed the mindset to make it a priority.*

If you want to achieve significant long-term benefits, then exercise needs to be made a part of your normal routine. Whether it consistently involves accumulating minutes during your busy workday, or is more structured by being scheduled, there must be a commitment to be more physically active, and it must be reaffirmed on a daily basis.

Get Out of Bed Running

Exercising is much like investing. Everyone knows that investing is a good thing to do. Many people do intend to invest regularly, but by the end of the month, after all the bills have been paid, there is usually not enough money remaining to put away in the stock market. People know they should exercise and really intend to do so, but by the end of the day, there usually is nothing physically left to enable them to get started.

The financial experts try to address this problem by urging people to invest with the first check of the month instead of the last—to pay themselves first, as it were. They are trying to make the act of investing such a priority that it is absolutely done on a regular basis. The same advice could be used to help people exercise. If possible, you should attempt to exercise first thing in the morning, when your energy level is high. Experts say this is the best time to exercise in order to boost your metabolism for the day. But, it is also the best time to ensure that you can develop and maintain a routine. Exercising later in the day is much harder to maintain because life frequently gets in the way. It always will be sacrificed in order to meet any number of life's distractions that tend to happen all the time.

A Rolling Stone Gathers No Moss

Getting anyone to develop a routine is much like trying to move a heavy boulder at the top of a large hill. Initially, it takes a lot of effort to get that boulder moving to the edge, but once it starts rolling down the hill, very little further effort is needed. Just so, once you start experiencing some of the rewards of being more physically active, you will become highly committed and motivated. The challenge is to get started.

Studies have been done to determine what interventions work best to get previously sedentary people to be more active. The Activity Counseling Trial (ACT) is one of the more respected of these studies. Conducted in primary health care settings, this trial examined different methods of motivating people to become more active or, thought of another way, different methods to get that boulder moving. It divided 800 patients into three groups and followed them over two years.[16]

Each group received different amounts of counseling during this time, ranging from eighteen minutes to nine hours. The results of the trial were interesting for several reasons. First, they showed that some people can change with little more than gentle encouragement. At the start of the trial, only 1 percent of the participants reported engaging in the daily recommended thirty minutes of physical activity. After two years and three brief counseling sessions (totaling eighteen minutes), upwards of 15 percent of the participants reported reaching that goal. More interesting, though, was the discovery that men and women responded differently to the interventions. For men, after receiving the initial advice, followed by brief reminders, it didn't matter how much more time or effort went into helping them achieve their goal. Statistically, they scored the same on objective measures of fitness regardless of the amount of counseling time. For women, the opposite proved true. As the amount of counseling increased to over three hours, they objectively showed more improvement in their fitness scores. This does not mean that men are faster learners. Rather, when presented with education about the benefits of increased physical activity, they either get it or they don't. More discussions proved to be fruitless. Men just need to be advised about the importance of being more active, and then periodically reminded.

In relation to this, it might be helpful to think about how wives try to get their husbands to do the things on their *honey-do* lists. Newly married wives spend a lot of time and effort trying to motivate their husbands to get to the things on the list, and they frequently get frustrated. The more experienced wives have come to learn that their husbands need to know what is on the list, and then be reminded occasionally. They come to realize that all the extra time and effort they might expend to motivate them is usually wasted energy. Their husbands either get it or they don't.

In the exercise arena, since women clearly did better as the counseling increased, this seems to coincide with the fact that women tend to be more socially wired. It is probable that success rates for getting women started and keeping them going on an exercise program would increase significantly if they enlisted the help of their friends. This help could take several forms, ranging from having friends as exercise partners to having the friends monitor their progress through phone calls, postcards, or e-mails.

Pain, No Gain—Avoiding Sports Injuries

The ACT study also provided insight into the potential risks of increased physical activity. Musculoskeletal injuries were by far the most frequently encountered adverse events. On average, approximately 30 percent of participants per year suffered a muscle or joint injury.[17]

It is important to be aware of this risk and to take measures to lessen it. Nothing stops momentum or breaks routine faster than an injury. Steps can be taken to lessen this risk, such as strict adherence to warm-up and cool-down periods, supervised workouts, and the regular use of protective equipment. Starting slow and gradually increasing intensity over time is probably most beneficial in preventing injuries.

There is also a small risk of developing a heart attack from unaccustomed increased physical exertion. It is estimated to be responsible for one death per year for every 15,000 men.[18]

This risk is greatest for the previously sedentary person who suddenly engages in high-intensity vigorous physical activity, such as shoveling snow after a major snowstorm. Overall, however, the potential risks from increasing physical activity seem to pale in comparison to the numerous health benefits that result from adopting such a change.

Every Eisenhower Needs a Patton

After World War I, two young Army officers frequently engaged in a friendly debate, arguing over what was most important for achieving victory on the battlefield. With his renowned attention to detail, Dwight D. Eisenhower believed success was all in the planning. George S. Patton, realizing that men have difficulty following plans when bullets are flying over their heads, claimed it was the leadership on the battlefields that ultimately won or lost the day. Both men went on to greatness and became highly decorated generals during World War II. Appropriately enough, Eisenhower, the planner, coordinated much of the war effort from his headquarters; Patton, the battlefield leader, made his fame on the front lines. Ironically, despite their differences in personality and philosophy, they needed each other. Without good planning, a headstrong general becomes nothing more than General Custer at Little Big Horn, massacred with all his men. Without good battlefield leadership, careful planners become nothing more than the French at the beginning of World War II, overrun by the Germans. If victory is to be had, planning and leadership must be equally important.

So it is with exercise. You need to not only plan your exercise routine, you need to be able to execute your plan as well. This is where much of the difficulty arises. Many would-be exercisers never make it past the planning phase. They are not disciplined enough to act on their plans. For these individuals, it is essential to find someone who acts as their Patton.

Whether it is a pushy friend, an assertive family member, or a personal trainer, you need strong encouragement to keep with the program. By taking time to develop this type of support system, you will be significantly increasing your chances of getting to your fitness plans, and staying with them as well.

Don't Ring the Bell

I made the mistake of watching the first part of the Demi Moore movie *GI Jane* with my six-year-old daughter. In this movie, the actress plays a naval officer attempting to be the first woman to successfully become a Navy SEAL. The first day appears especially brutal as the sleep-deprived soldiers in full-battle gear are doing push-ups in the cold ocean surf. As night approaches and the soldiers are eagerly awaiting their desperately needed rest, the officer in charge of training—in an effort to break their spirit—informs them that the first day doesn't end until somebody quits. As might be expected, quitting is the last thing these fanatical soldiers would want to do. They push themselves well beyond physical exhaustion until they can barely stand. It is only when their mental will is broken that they take the walk of shame to the bell in the middle of the complex and ring it, signifying they have (embarrassingly) quit. My mistake occurred when I bragged to my daughter that I would never ring that bell. Two weeks later, after I had again begun exercising, my daughter watched as I struggled to do sit-ups. I would like to say I was finishing my hundredth sit-up, but it was probably closer to my thirtieth, when I collapsed back to the floor and said I couldn't do any more. Imagine how I felt when my daughter teased, "You're ringing the bell, Daddy, you're ringing the bell." It seems I had found my Patton.

Exercise is much more a mental challenge than a physical one. You have to strengthen your mind before you can strengthen your body. This is manifested by mentally developing a commitment to improve your body and reaffirming this commitment on a daily basis. Be an inspiration to others by living this commitment. Whatever you do, don't quit trying; don't ring that bell.

Exercise Tips

1. Throughout your day, accumulate at least thirty minutes of moderate-intensity physical activity that equals the exertion needed for a brisk walk.

2. Three times a week, attempt to schedule more structured exercise.

3. Pay yourself first by exercising in the morning before life gets in the way.

4. Enlist a pushy friend to be your exercise partner.

5. Encourage others to regularly ask about your exercise routine.

6. The best way to avoid injuries is by starting slow and gradually increasing the intensity of the workout over time. (FYI: Approximately 30 percent of exercisers sustain an injury during the year, which stops their routine temporarily and sometimes permanently.)

7. Pick a day to get started, and when that day comes, stick to the commitment and get started.

6

BLOOD PRESSURE

You're just like everybody else
You'll come to a place where
You'll have to answer to your own pressure.
—BILLY JOEL, *PRESSURE*

My first car was a 1967 black Plymouth Fury. It was a big car, measuring over eighteen feet from bumper to bumper. It sat four, comfortably, across the backseat, and it closely resembled the Batmobile. The car oozed character. I would have looked fairly impressive driving that car to school in 1967, but I didn't own the car at that time. In fact, I wasn't even born yet. I'm fairly certain I didn't look quite as impressive driving that car to school in 1987. Despite the fact that I could have applied for an antique license plate, I loved that car, though, to be completely honest, I should say, I *initially* loved that car.

The honeymoon period came to an end after the car had had continual breakdowns. At least once a month, I would get stranded somewhere with a car that wouldn't start. I wish I could say I had taken this opportunity to learn all about car engines. However, it would be more accurate to say I only learned enough not to be laughed at by the person who came to my rescue. I had gotten real good at opening the hood of the car and looking seriously at the engine for a few minutes. I would nod my head several times, as if I were getting close to detecting what the problem might be. Eventually, after enough time had elapsed, I would come to the conclusion that I'd better start looking for a pay phone if I ever wanted to get home.

My greatest frustration resulted from the fact that there was rarely any forewarning of an impending problem. The car would seem to be running well. It would maintain its pick-up. There would be no funny noises. It would wait for the most inopportune time, as for example when I was out on a date, and it would just quit. It should not have been unexpected for a twenty-year-old car to have some mechanical problems. (I wonder if there is a conversion chart for car years to human years as they have for dogs.) In retrospect, I have to take some of the responsibility for the mechanical failures. I was not the best person at preventive car maintenance. (I'm still not.) I always used the cheapest gas; I rarely changed the oil; and, frankly, I was scared to take it in for a tune-up for fear they might not give it back to me.

Car-engine troubles and blood-pressure problems seem very analogous. In both cases, there are usually no obvious outward signs that something may be wrong. Just as I was unaware that my car engine was not performing well, most people with high blood pressure have no idea that their pressure is high. When an engine is not running efficiently, it, too, gradually starts to build higher pressures. As a result, the parts that comprise the engine start to wear out faster.

If you consistently maintain higher pressures in your system, your parts, too, will begin to wear down. While with the car engine, the talk is about problems with pistons and cylinders, in the human body the talk is about problems with the brain, heart, and kidneys. Just as the car engine eventually shuts downs, after years of higher pressures the human body also experiences its own breakdowns in the form of heart attacks, kidney failures, and strokes. Preventive car maintenance can prevent or delay mechanical problems and the same can be said for dealing with blood-pressure problems. Developing a better understanding about what constitutes preventive blood-pressure measures, is what this chapter is all about.

A Fate Worse than Death

Imagine being at a dinner party, when all of a sudden you can no longer express yourself. Your mind is working OK. You know what you want to say, but, when you try to say it, the words don't come out right. Imagine the panic you begin to feel. You get up to go, but you forget how to put on your coat. Not understanding what is happening, people start smiling at you, thinking you might have drunk too much. You know you need to get to a hospital, but your frustration only heightens because you can't tell someone to take you. Imagine the fear as you think this might be permanent. These are some of the more common symptoms people experience when they are having a stroke. If you can truly imagine them, then you will begin to appreciate why blood-pressure management is important.

Unfortunately, many at-risk people don't even know they *are* at risk. It is estimated that 50 million Americans have high blood pressure, of which, more than 15 million are not aware they have it. It certainly has earned its nickname, the silent killer.[1]

Many studies have shown a direct relationship between blood-pressure control and cardiovascular events, such as heart attacks and strokes. These studies have consistently demonstrated that the greater the blood pressure, the greater the risk.[2]

Fortunately, this risk can be modified by controlling pressure with changes in lifestyle and, possibly, with medications. The challenge is getting people to adopt these changes when they don't feel bad.

Why Is the Blood Pressurized?

Many people do not appreciate the complexity the body has acquired in attempting to regulate its blood pressure. Most know that 120 over 80 is fairly normal, but they don't understand how much goes into actually developing that number.

As a candle continually needs oxygen to stay alight, every cell in your body needs oxygen to stay alive. Getting that oxygen to the cells is the main reason why your blood has a pressure. In order to achieve this, your body transports blood in either arteries or veins. Arteries take your blood, with its fresh supply of oxygen, away from the heart, while veins bring your blood, with its depleted oxygen supply, back toward your heart, going through your lungs to resupply with oxygen.

Anatomically, there are rather significant differences between arteries and veins. The two most important revolve around the fact that arteries have muscles in their walls and they are in a pressurized system. The ability of arteries to narrow or expand, depending on whether the muscular layer contracts or relaxes, affords your body much needed flexibility to possibly divert blood flow to areas where it is most needed. By having a pressurized system, your body is able to circulate the blood in such a way that it can continually resupply with oxygen. The top pressure in this system occurs immediately *after* each heartbeat, when blood is pumped out from your heart to the rest of your body. This number is called the systolic pressure (aka the top number). As your heart is refilling, the pressure in the system begins dropping. The lowest level of pressure occurs immediately *before* your next heartbeat and is called the diastolic pressure (aka the bottom number).

It is generally accepted that the height of your blood pressure is the product of two basic factors—cardiac output and total peripheral resistance. Cardiac output is equivalent to the amount and rate at which your blood is pumped out of your heart. This, in turn, is affected by your heart rate, the strength of your heartbeat, and the total amount of blood in your body. Peripheral resistance is present because, as the arteries get farther and farther from your heart and into the peripheral areas, they get smaller and smaller, making it more difficult for the blood to continue to pass.

Your body has evolved many ways to exert influence on its own pressure. It often releases multiple hormones to either increase or decrease your pressure depending on the circumstances. It also has direct nerve connections, which provide more immediate effects on your arteries. Regionally, it is able to exert local control over a particular artery, by making it responsive to such things as the acidity of your blood, the oxygen content of nearby tissues, or the smaller hormones released by the wall of the artery itself. Much of this process falls under the direct supervision of your kidneys, which influence blood pressure by controlling blood volume and releasing hormones that affect peripheral resistance. It is important for you to appreciate this complexity of the blood-pressure system in order to best understand the multiple, different approaches that can be utilized to potentially correct it.

Blood Pressure—A Moving Target

Inherent in this complexity is the fact that your blood pressure frequently fluctuates throughout the day. It is a moving target, which can change literally minute to minute. Your blood pressure can be elevated if you're sick, if you're upset, if you're stressed, or if you're in pain. It can be elevated if you were hurried getting to the doctor's office, or if the doctor had been running late. Many over-the-counter medications, such as anti-inflammatory drugs and decongestants, can raise blood pressure, and they often go unreported by people who don't consider them medications.

Experts continually remind physicians not to overreact to one reading, but rather encourage them to look for trends in multiple readings over time, before adding or changing therapy. It can be frightening to think that treatment decisions might be based on one moment of your day, when so many other variables could possibly be playing a role.

Home Blood Pressure Monitors—Fact or Fiction?

Equally frightening to physicians are the many difficulties associated with blood-pressure-measuring devices (otherwise known as manometers). In order to correctly manage your blood pressure, a physician must have some confidence that the data that he is analyzing is accurate. An Italian physician, Dr. Scipione Riva-Rocci, was the first to devise a blood-pressure device, and it was brought to the United States in 1901 by Dr. Harvey Cushing.[3,4]

Over the years, the mercury manometer has come to be the gold standard for blood-pressure measurement in physicians' offices as well as in hospitals. There are numerous studies documenting its accuracy when used correctly. Problems can arise if the wrong cuff size is used (too small a cuff can give a falsely elevated reading), if the person taking the reading is inattentive, or if there is a preconceived bias as to what the blood pressure should be (which happens more than might be expected).

These reliable and accurate mercury devices started being systematically replaced in June 1998. In response to the increasing concern over the toxic effects of mercury exposure, the Environmental Protection Agency (EPA), developed regulations to limit as much mercury waste from hospitals as possible by 2005.[5]

As a result of these regulations, aneroid devices have become increasingly utilized. In these devices, the liquid mercury, normally present in the classic blood-pressure machine, has been replaced by a metallic spring. Not surprisingly, as the metallic spring ages, the accuracy of these devices tends to wane, with no obvious signal that this may be happening. They can conceivably be reporting faulty data for months, without anyone suspecting any problems. It is imperative that these devices be calibrated regularly to ensure their accuracy, but whether this is routinely done or not would vary from institution to institution. A study from 1991 found that, at one particular university hospital, 80 percent of the aneroid blood-pressure devices had been inaccurate.[6]

As more Americans are becoming health conscious, the sales of home blood-pressure monitors are soaring. The mercury and aneroid devices are classified as *manual* machines, and they require a person with a stethoscope to operate. The home devices are generally *automated,* designed for self-use. In theory, the home monitors provide an excellent opportunity to provide a clearer picture of the overall trend in blood-pressure readings. In practice, these notoriously unreliable machines have made many physicians hesitant to use the data they supply.

There are hundreds of different brands of blood-pressure monitors sold worldwide. Most experts would agree that finger and wrist devices should be avoided, as they tend to be the least accurate. With regard to the upper arm monitors, there can be rather significant variation in the quality of these devices. In an effort to address this well-known problem, patients often attempt to test the accuracy of their monitors at doctors' offices, and all too often they leave disappointed by how poorly their machines performed. Fortunately, there is still hope for the informed consumer who can start making selections of devices based on *validation* results.

In 1987, the American Association for the Advancement of Medical Instrumentation (AAMI) published a protocol for evaluating the accuracy of blood-pressure machines. In 1990, the British Hypertension Society (BHS) developed its own protocol, and together the AAMI and the BHS have gained international acclaim for their ability to assess the accuracy of devices.[7,8]

Fearing that they couldn't meet the protocol's high standards, most companies have chosen not to have their blood pressure machines evaluated by these societies. The machines that *do* get passing grades from these societies would therefore be the most desirable monitors to purchase.

The White-Coat Effect—Real or Imagined?

With the increasing availability of these home blood-pressure monitors, the white-coat effect (aka white-coat hypertension) is coming to the forefront in many people's thinking. It is estimated that as many as 25 percent of all people experience white-coat hypertension. This is a condition where a person has an elevated blood pressure in the doctor's office, but consistently has normal blood pressure when measured at home. Most experts would agree this is a real phenomenon. It was first documented in 1940, and its existence has been proven in numerous studies ever since.[9,10,11]

The real question is not whether white-coat hypertension exists, but rather if it should be treated? On the one hand, some researchers believe the white-coat effect is fairly benign and not associated with any serious cardiovascular problems. They argue there is no documented proof that this sudden and brief surge in blood pressure has any negative long-term side effects. They also caution physicians about unnecessarily overtreating patients with potentially dangerous and costly medications. On the other hand, there are an equal number of researchers who disagree completely, and argue that the white-coat effect is associated with some long-term problems, and should be treated.[12,13]

It is probably safe to assume that people with high blood pressure only during periods of heightened stress, such as in a doctor's office, will have less long-term complications than those who have elevated pressures all the time. The question becomes, "How much less?" At present, it is most important to attempt to identify who might potentially have this condition, and it can be done by having them wear a blood-pressure monitor for twenty-four hours, a procedure known as an ambulatory twenty-four-hour blood-pressure test. Given its cost and limited availability, however, it is much more practical to have people check their own pressures with home monitors. If a consistent discrepancy between home and office blood-pressure readings is found, then the diagnosis of white-coat hypertension can be made. In these instances, it is usually best to maximize non-medication approaches, such as encouraging weight loss, restricting salt, reducing stress, and promoting exercise. More research is needed to determine whether physicians need to be more aggressive in treating this undeniable condition.

JNC VII—How Low Should It Go?

Given the many complexities of blood-pressure management, a rather elaborate collaboration of experts, organizations, and agencies was created to assist physicians in the proper handling of blood-pressure problems. Officially known as the National High Blood Pressure Education Program (NHBPEP) Coordinating Committee (quite a mouthful), this association regularly releases its recommendations under the title of Joint National Committee (JNC) Reports. These JNC reports are considered the gold standard for the latest approach to hypertension. The most current of these reports is the Seventh Report of the Joint National Committee, which was released in May 2003. Prior to this, the 1997 recommendations from JNC VI had been in effect. As enough new evidence accumulates, the JNC will continue to update its standards to stay aligned with the current thinking of the day.

There were some rather significant changes in the JNC VII report. For starters, it seems to have answered the long debated question: Which is the more important number? It appears that the systolic (top) reading, is the most predictive of future cardiovascular problems, at least for people fifty years or older.[13]

More importantly, JNC VII simplified the classification system for blood-pressure management. Normal blood pressure has been redefined as a systolic pressure below 120 mm Hg. A new category of *prehypertension* has been created to refer to those with systolic blood pressures between 120 and 139 mm Hg. Previously considered normal, these people should be counseled on the benefits of lifestyle modifications, as they are considered at higher risk for cardiovascular events. Stage 1 hypertension and stage 2 hypertension refer to people with systolic pressures greater than 140 and 160 mm Hg, respectively. Stage 1 hypertension generally requires at least one blood-pressure medication, while stage 2 usually requires at least two medications. This new classification system underscores the point that, as the blood pressure gets higher, so too does the risk of complications.

Minimize Medications—Maximize Lifestyle Changes

Lifestyle modifications should be emphasized in anyone who consistently is found to have blood-pressure readings greater than 120 mm Hg. These modifications are thought to generally include losing weight, stopping smoking, limiting caffeine and sodium intake, increasing exercise, and avoiding alcohol. The effects these changes might bring are varied, and much depends on the individual circumstances. Generally speaking, though, weight loss is probably the best way to lower pressure. Some studies have reported as much as a 20 mm Hg decrease in blood pressure with every 10 kilogram decrease in weight.[14]

More simply, for the overweight person it would be reasonable to expect that, for every pound lost, there would be a corresponding drop of one point in their blood pressure reading. It is important to try and maximize these lifestyle changes in order to avoid having to take medications, as those used to lower blood pressure tend to be permanent additions to the bathroom shelves—it is very unusual to stop blood-pressure medications once they've been started. Frequently, they can be changed to other medications, but they are rarely ever out-and-out stopped. Other drawbacks to these medications include:

- They can be very difficult to remember to take because there is no immediate positive effect from their usage.

- They have many potential side effects.

- They are costly.

- They can have limited effectiveness, with the result that most people need two or more of them to reach their goal of lowered pressure.

In sum, maximize lifestyle changes to minimize medications. You'll find that the health benefits from this mindset are incalculable.[15]

The ABCDs of Blood-Pressure Medications

There is a wide array of blood-pressure medications for which textbooks have been written. It might be helpful to know there are four basic groups from which these medications are normally drawn. They start with the first four letters of the alphabet: ACE inhibitors (and the closely related ARB agents); beta blockers; calcium channel blockers; and diuretics (water pills). Each of these classes has its strengths and weaknesses. And each has its own risk of side effects. The JNC VII report stressed that most people with uncomplicated hypertension should be on diuretics, "either alone or combined with drugs from other classes."[16]

Depending on pre-existing conditions, medication from any class may be appropriate as a starting point. Many people are on drugs from two, three, or four of these subclasses, underscoring the point that controlling blood pressure can be very difficult. As they age, the challenge for doctors often becomes keeping them on only one or two of these drugs. It is important to remember, though, that by maintaining people near their blood pressure goal, they will be receiving some very tangible benefits. Statistically, studies have shown that they will be 35 to 40 percent less likely to have a stroke, 20 to 25 percent less likely to have a heart attack, and 50 percent less likely to have heart failure.[17]

Sooner or Later

Subconsciously, everyone does a cost assessment weighing potential future medical problems against the effort needed to possibly prevent them. This analysis can prove difficult, when dealing with blood pressure. Generally, it doesn't make you feel bad, when your pressure is high. This makes taking action to treat it a hard pill to swallow. Also, there is a disconnect in time, usually extending over years, between the onset of high blood pressure and the time an adverse event occurs, if one ever does.

If these problems are not enough, there are other obstacles impeding proper management of the condition. Acquiring accurate results is one challenge, establishing a definite trend is another. There are so many variables that can artificially raise pressure that sometimes the task can seem overwhelming. Despite these impediments, however, the high incidence of heart attacks, congestive heart failure, and strokes in today's world demands that more time and effort go into education, so these hurdles can be overcome.

After reviewing the JNC VII report, I was most surprised by the statement that reads "individuals who are normotensive at fifty-five years of age have a 90 percent lifetime risk for developing hypertension."[18]

It would seem that everyone is destined to fight this battle at some point. Given a choice on how to approach the problem, some will take an active role, adopting lifestyle changes, taking medications regularly, checking readings routinely, in order to lessen the negative impact of high blood pressure. Then, there are others who will take the opposite approach, refusing to change behavior, infrequently taking medications, and becoming resigned to the philosophy—what will be, will be.

Eventually, though, whether you want it to or not, there will come a time in your life when you will have to live with the earlier decisions you made regarding your pressure.

Blood Pressure Tips

1. Be sure to get your blood pressure checked any time the opportunity presents itself, especially if it is done with a stethoscope. Write down the results.

2. If you or anyone in your family has problems with blood pressure, invest in an AAMI/BHS-validated home monitoring system. Then, get it rechecked in your doctor's office.

3. Look for the recommendations of the Joint National Committee or JNC, which sets the standards for blood-pressure management. Be aware that they are separate from the drug industry and are, as a result, unbiased.

4. Your blood pressure may be elevated normally in response to stress, illness, pain, and other medications. Pay particular attention to anti-inflammatory medications, as they can often cause blood pressure to be elevated.

5. Maximize non-medication therapies if your blood pressure is trending upwards. If you do regular aerobic exercise, your blood pressure will drop about eight points. If you're overweight and lose some weight, your blood pressure will drop almost a point for each pound lost. And if you adhere to a diet low in salt, low in alcohol, and high in fiber, you can lower your blood pressure by several points as well.

6. Some people need three or four medications to control their blood pressure. If you are taking medications, be sure to have an updated list in your wallet or pocketbook. Know that there are four major classes of blood-pressure medications—ACE inhibitors or ARB agents; beta blockers; calcium channel blockers; and diuretics—and know which of these classes you are taking.

7. Much like the ocean that causes beach erosion over time, the effects of high blood pressure also occur gradually over many years. One high tide, or one high blood-pressure reading, will not be likely to have much impact on the big picture—it's the overall trend that's most important.

7

NATURE'S ROLE IN HEALTH

Study nature, love nature, stay close to nature.
It will never fail you.
—FRANK LLOYD WRIGHT (*UNSOURCED*)

When my wife was twelve, she spent the summer at the beach, working in an ice cream parlor. Her training lasted all of about thirty seconds, and it consisted of her boss showing her how to hold a cone underneath the ice cream dispensing machine. On her first day, her boss informed her that he needed to run a few errands and left her unattended in the store. He reassured her it shouldn't be that busy, and promised to be back in a few hours.

Her first customer was a woman requesting soft serve vanilla ice cream dipped in chocolate. Well, she hadn't been debriefed on the dipping process, so, in a bit of a panic, she cleverly came up with the excuse that the dipping machine was broken. Not wanting to be sugar deprived, the customer requested jimmies (sprinkles) as her next topping of choice. Equally unfamiliar with the jimmying process, and fairly certain that the woman wouldn't fall for the broken-machine line again, my wife decided to fake it. Unfortunately, she couldn't stop the ice cream from falling off the cone as she attempted to apply the jimmies. Eventually, she presented the woman with a sloppy, dripping cone that looked more like someone picked it up off the floor than made it special for her. Adding further insult to injury, she then made the poor woman pay, or overpay, as she later found out, for this less than ideal ice cream delight. Scores of ice cream seekers filled the store that day. My wife desperately tried to keep up with the demand, and she basically learned as she went along.

It was this exact sensation of lack of preparedness that I experienced early in my career, when I began treating patients who were more interested in avoiding, rather than taking medicines, to improve their health. My training, which was fairly standard for most primary care physicians, consisted of only a few voluntary lectures on alternative treatments, most of which were poorly attended. I had no formal training on supplements, and no formal nutritional training that would have highlighted which foods possess health benefits. Basically, I underestimated the demand that would be thrust upon me, not realizing just how many people were interested in these topics, and, like my wife, I, had to learn on the run.

You, too, have probably had a similar sensation of learning on the run when it came to finding out answers to questions in these areas. Most of your knowledge will likely have come from self-study, acquired from reading books, talking with friends, or surfing the Internet.

As my wife eventually became proficient at serving ice cream—she still makes a mean sundae—I eventually became proficient in counseling regarding natural alternatives that would benefit my patients' overall health. From my own self-study, this is what I learned.

RED, BROWN, GREEN FLAVONOIDS, AND OMEGA-3 TO THE RESCUE

Red, Red Wine . . .

In America, the term *French paradox* first appeared during a 1991 *60 Minutes* broadcast. It referred to the surprisingly low incidence of heart disease in France, a country known for its intake of cheeses, chocolates, and other rich foods. Many credited the French people's love of red wine as the source of their longevity. Thus was born the red wine craze that dominated the 1990s and beyond.

How much did red wine consumption actually increase in America? Following that news show in 1991, almost to the exact month, red wine bottles started flying off the shelves in liquor stores across the country. Throughout the 1990s, red wine sales increased by over 125 percent.[1]

People were choosing red wine because they thought it was healthy for them, because they knew it was trendy, and because they liked it—a classic win-win-win scenario for the wine industry. But the question remained, did red wine possess any extra health benefits, making it worthy of all the special attention it was receiving?

To answer this question, it may be helpful to think of wine as containing both an alcohol-based component in the form of ethanol and a plant-based component in the form of polyphenols. Numerous studies have demonstrated that alcohol, when consumed in moderation, reduces heart attacks, strokes, and overall mortality. The estimates may vary, but most studies report a 30 to 50 percent reduction in heart attacks in people who admit to moderate alcohol intake. This reduction has been seen with red wine, white wine, spirits, and beer.[2,3]

There are also studies showing that one to two alcoholic drinks per day may reduce your risk of developing diabetes, and may even help maintain your cognitive function as you get older.[4,5]

So, as strange as it may sound, drinking alcohol may actually be healthy for you. But, the important phrase to remember is *when used in moderation*. This is easier said than done. What does drinking in moderation really mean? As a general rule, it means one drink per day for women, and one to two drinks per day for men. Drink, of course, is not defined in gallons, but in ounces. Officially, one drink equals a 12-ounce beer, a 5-ounce glass of wine, or 1.5-ounces of 80-proof spirits.

When you exceed this one to two drink per day minimum, and this is very easy to do, you lose all the potential health benefits, and you start acquiring all the torments that predictably walk hand in hand with chronic alcohol use. So, you need to be careful, especially if you have a family history of alcoholism. If this is the case, you should stay away from alcohol altogether.

As the studies have shown, it is clear that red wine has some definite health benefits from its alcohol content alone, but what about its polyphenol content? Do the plant-derived polyphenol compounds found in red wine offer additional health benefits, making it more desirable for you to choose when you sit down for your evening meal?

Red wine, because it is fermented with its skin, has a much higher level of polyphenols than white wine. These polyphenols are compounds acquired from the skin, the seed, and the pulp of the grape. Generally, there are four major types of poyphenols. These include resveratrol, flavonoids, proanthocyanidins, and anthocyanins. Together these compounds are thought to possess healing properties by acting like natural antioxidants.

When you bite into an apple, the exposed fruit turns brown when it encounters oxygen. In a sense, it has become oxidized. A similar reaction occurs inside your body when oxygen interacts with your various cells. Although critical for existence, oxygen can have some unwanted effects. It can activate your bad cholesterol, or LDL, making it more dangerous and more likely to form plaque. It also contributes to the formation of free radicals, compounds that can injure other cells in your body. Antioxidants are able to neutralize this damage done by oxygen, and thus make you healthier. The concept that polyphenols are a rich source of antioxidants has led to rampant speculation that red wine is healthier for you.

Even among red wines, though, the polyphenol content is highly variable. It depends on the type of grape used, the climate during which the grapes were grown, and the manner in which the grapes were allowed to ferment into wine. Generally speaking, the higher the polyphenol content, the greater perceived benefit you would receive. There is also great variability in the types of polyphenols among red wines. Some may have higher quantities of resveratrol, while others have higher amounts of flavonoids. This has led to a great debate as to which polyphenol, and by extension, which red wine, would be healthiest for you.

In 2000, this speculation that resveratrol was the answer became fever-pitched. This compound is typically found in the skin of some grapes, and acts as the grape's natural defense against fungus. As a result, it is found more commonly in grapes grown in climates that are cold and rainy, conditions where fungus tends to flourish. Touted as a wonder drug by most researchers, resveratrol seemed to possess anti-aging properties, even going so far as to extend the lifespan of obese mice. (Yes, even mice have obesity problems.) Many people started drinking Pinot Noir wines because they were known to have high levels of this compound. Unfortunately, you would have to drink hundreds of bottles of wine a day to equal the amount of resveratrol that was fed to the obese mice, making many question whether it has much impact in humans, and whether it truly was the answer.[6,7]

Resveratrol, in addition to being in the skin of grapes, is also found in blueberries, mulberries, and in some peanuts. While it may not be present in sufficient amounts in wine to exert a beneficial effect, many people have chosen to take it in higher amounts as a supplement. Since resveratrol only began to be seriously studied in the year 2000, there is insufficient data to determine its long-term effectiveness in humans when taken as an isolated supplement. The major question is whether it can get absorbed when taken this way, and if so, will it still deliver the desired impact. To date, it appears safe and very promising, but further study is needed to determine just how safe and beneficial it really is.

In the November 2006 issue of *Nature,* the French paradox was re-evaluated, and thought to be more a regional phenomenon. The increased longevity didn't involve all of France, but rather seemed to concentrate in Southwest France (including the Italian island of Sardinia).[8]

The wines made in these areas tended to be bitter, with higher levels of condensed tannins. These regions believed in classic winemaking, allowing the grapes to ferment for four weeks, rather than the usual one week, providing ample time for all the polyphenols to be absorbed from the skin of the grape. Contemporary winemaking intentionally tries to remove these tannins to get rid of the bitter taste. It is probable that the red wines with the highest polyphenol content across the board, including all the different types, such as flavonoids and procyanidins, will offer you the greatest health benefit.

Ironically, Americans started drinking red wine in the 1990s for its perceived health benefit, yet the red wine most Americans drink is probably no healthier than other alcoholic beverages, since the majority of its polyphenols are intentionally removed to get rid of the bitter taste. If you are choosing red wine for its health benefits, remember that bitter is better. Try choosing a full-bodied Cabernet Sauvignon or Pinot Noir at your next dinner party, and remember the toast: "To your health."

Death by Chocolate—Fact or Fiction?

If you are like most people, you probably feel guilty when you empty that box of chocolates you receive on special occasions. With recent advances, you may not need to feel so bad. There has been a major movement promoting the health benefits of dark chocolate during the past ten years. This has been fueled by the discovery that cocoa, the parent plant of chocolate, contains large amounts of flavonoids.

As you saw with wine, flavonoids are plant-derived substances that seem to possess healing properties. Plants make flavonoids to repair themselves from environmental damage. When consumed by humans, they are thought to act much like antioxidants, lessening injury to blood vessels, and lowering blood pressure.

A real life example of this effect can be seen by studying the Kuna Indians of Central America. Their incidence of heart disease, high blood pressure, and cancer is so low that many have turned to their diet for possible explanations. Researchers now believe it is their daily consumption of three to four pure cocoa drinks that accounts for their incredible longevity.

The Kuna Indians are a fascinating study group. Half their members became urbanized, adopting the city life of Central Americans, while half remained isolated in the jungle, maintaining their tribal culture. The group that migrated to the city developed similar incidences of heart disease to their city counterparts. But the group that remained isolated in the jungle had a much lower incidence of heart problems, high blood pressure, and cancer. Given that they shared the same genetics, it became clear that an environmental change was responsible for the difference. This is why their diet was closely examined, as it was the biggest change in the environment, and this is how they found that the cocoa drink, and by extension, dark chocolate, was affording tribe members a distinct health advantage.

Researchers even went further trying to find out how the cocoa drink might be exerting a positive effect. They discovered that the tribal group had much higher levels of nitric oxide in their urine. This is a compound known to help blood vessels stay healthy by keeping them maximally dilated and free of plaque. It is thought to be the reason why the cocoa drink is good for you.[9]

Hernando Cortez brought a similar cocoa drink back with him to Europe in the 1500s after he conquered the Aztecs. The problem was it was too bitter for most people to drink. (As with wine, bitter appears to be better when it comes to the healthiness of the foods you eat or drink.) It was only when they added cane sugar that the drink became appealing to all, nullifying, in the process, many of its innate benefits.

As chocolate becomes more processed, much of its flavonoid content gets stripped away, leaving a product loaded with sugars, fats, and other additives. The sugar is the biggest problem, as it significantly increases the calorie content.

Are you able to get the same health benefits by eating dark chocolate on a daily basis? This is a difficult question to answer. As with red wine, where you would have to drink upward of hundreds of bottles of wine a day to achieve the same blood levels of resveratrol fed to the obese mice, the Kuna Indians regularly consume about 900 milligrams of flavonoids a day, which would translate into a very large amount of dark chocolate.

That being said, the chocolate industry, excited by the recent studies, has been experimenting with ways to make their product healthier by increasing their flavonoid content. Some of the premium-grade chocolates have higher cocoa contents, and use only cocoa butter as their saturated fat. This is important because cocoa butter is the only saturated fat that has a neutral effect on your cholesterol. (As a general rule, you should always avoid all saturated and trans fats.) Cocoa butter melts just below body temperature, and it is is responsible for the wonderful sensation of chocolate melting in your mouth.

There have been several studies trying to demonstrate the benefits from daily intake of commercial chocolate products. Most of these studies have either too few participants or too short a time frame to draw any definite conclusions. Several studies have shown that daily consumption of small amounts of dark chocolate can lower blood pressure by four to five points. With regard to preventing heart disease, there is only limited data at present, and more studies need to be performed before widespread recommendations can be made.[10]

In January 2006, researchers believed they had found the secret ingredient in flavonoids that was providing all the health benefit in cocoa. Epicatechin, as it is called, is believed responsible for improving blood flow through arteries, by increasing nitric oxide production. In subjects who consumed the pure cocoa drink, their blood levels of epicatechin were found to be very high, as were their levels of nitric oxide in the urine. Whether these effects will be seen if epicatechin is taken as a supplement is not yet known, but preliminary data is certainly promising.[11]

As a general rule of thumb, if you take a small amount of premium grade dark chocolate with a high cocoa content once daily, you will likely receive at least some health benefit. As with wine, bitter is better, and less is more. Take a small piece of dark chocolate, and smile, knowing that this may actually be healthy for you.

Gimme All Your Omega-3s . . . Go Fish

In the 1970s, researchers discovered a situation they had a difficult time explaining. The prevailing thought had always been that a diet high in fat would invariably lead to premature atherosclerosis and early heart disease. This theory was supported by all the studies, and seemed to apply to people from all walks of life. Then, a problem arose. When scientists began studying the Eskimos living in Greenland, known as the Inuits, they noticed an intriguing fact. Despite consuming a diet very high in fat, equal to or greater than the average Western diet, these Eskimos were found to have a very low incidence of heart disease. In fact, they were found to have a very low incidence of other diseases as well, such as diabetes, psoriasis, and rheumatoid arthritis. Perplexed, researchers wondered what could possibly be causing this phenomenon. They quickly concluded that the answer must lie in the type of fat that the Eskimos were consuming. Their fat was primarily obtained from coldwater fish, and it contained a new (to them) substance that came to be known as omega-3 fish oil. This was the secret ingredient affording all the health benefits, and this was the start of an amazing story, a story whose significance might actually be bigger than the initial researchers ever imagined, a story whose chapters are still being written, even decades later.[12]

Since their discovery in the 1970s, omega-3 fatty acids have been on a roller-coaster ride of scientific inquiry. They have been the subject of over 4,000 medical studies, and they have been considered as possible treatment options for close to a 100 different diseases. How could one compound have such a broad impact? The answer to this question lies in its unique role as the counterbalancing agent in the inflammatory cascade.

The inflammatory cascade is your body's emergency response system. Imagine, if you will, that your house is on fire. Soon after the 911 call, police cars will be diverting traffic from your street to contain the fire; firemen with axes will be knocking through your doors, and breaking your windows to gain better access to the flames, and water will be continuously pumped into your house from the fire engines on your street.

In a nutshell, this is how the inflammatory cascade works in your body when it perceives its own crisis. Whenever you injure your knee, twist your ankle, break a bone, or accidentally cut yourself, this cascade gets instantly turned on. As a result, you will soon see the hallmarks of inflammation—pain, redness, warmth, and swelling. In our analogy, the pain would be the 911 call alerting you that you have a problem. The redness and warmth would be the result of the firemen, in this case, your inflammatory cells, causing damage as they try to fix the problem. And the swelling would be the result of the increased blood flow to the area, your body's equivalent of water being continuously pumped to the fire.

In order for your body's inflammatory cascade to work properly, it needs its special tools, the inflammatory compounds, available and ready to go. Your body cannot make these compounds on its own. Rather it must acquire certain essential fatty acids from your diet and make these inflammatory compounds, using these fatty acids as building blocks. The type of fatty acid the body needs to accomplish this goal is the omega-6, not the omega-3 fatty acid. Omega-6 fatty acids are extremely prevalent in the Western diet—they are found in many baked goods, fried foods, grains, and vegetable oils.

By consuming a diet high in the omega-6 fatty acids, it is thought that you are promoting inflammation. In essence, you will be creating a bigger and bigger emergency response team, one which may be more likely to respond even when there is no crisis. This is the root cause of *many* diseases, and explains why consuming the wrong type of fatty acid may be really bad for you.

After the fire in your house has been extinguished, you can only imagine the mess you would find. There would be physical damage from the fire and smoke, and there would be water everywhere. It would require an extensive clean-up effort. As there is an inflammatory cascade, there is also an anti-inflammatory cascade. This complementary system is designed to clean up the mess by limiting the damage caused by inflammation. This anti-inflammatory system also makes its own compounds from fatty acids absorbed from your diet. These anti-inflammatory fatty acids are known as the omega-3 compounds. Their consumption helps keep the inflammatory system in check. This is the proposed basis for all the health benefits from fish oils, and this is why there have been so many disease treatments connected with their use.

So, omega-6 fatty acids are pro-inflammatory, and omega-3 fatty acids are anti-inflammatory. In addition to promoting these opposite functions, these fatty acids share the same equipment in the body that is used to make their corresponding inflammatory and anti-inflammatory compounds. This shared equipment, then, becomes a valued commodity for which the omega-6 and omega-3 actively compete. Think of these two agents trying to hail down the same cab. It becomes clear that the ratio of omega-6 to omega-3 in your diet will ultimately determine who will consistently get the cab more often. If this ratio favors the omega-6 fatty acids, the scales will be tipped toward more inflammation in your body (and more disease). If this ratio favors omega-3 fatty acids, as seen in the Eskimos of Greenland, then the scales will lean toward less inflammation (and better health).

The Western diet, derived primarily from grain and grain-fed animals, very much favors the omega-6 fatty acids, with typical ratios ranging from 20:1 to 30:1 (omega-6:omega-3). Ideally, it should be closer to 4:1 to reach a proper balance between the inflammatory and anti-inflammatory forces.[13,14]

An important point to remember is that inflammation, in and of itself, is not bad. If there is a fire in your house, you want the emergency response team to be there. It is when the team is there in excess, as when you have a barbecue in your backyard, that problems start to arise.

Another item worth mentioning is that omega-3 fatty acids can be derived from both plants and fish. Alpha-linolenic acid (ALA) is the main plant-derived omega-3. It is found in certain vegetable oils, like canola, flaxseed, and soybean, and it is also found in some nuts, like walnuts. Eicosapentaenoic acid (EPA) and docosahexaenoic acid (DHA) are the omega-3 fish oils found almost exclusively in coldwater fish, such as herring, mackerel, salmon, and sardines. Although the plant-derived and fish-derived fatty acids are both omega-3, they each offer their own unique health benefits, and should be viewed as completely different sets of compounds. All things being considered, the fish oils offer the most health benefits, and certainly have the better data when it comes to evidence supporting their use.

When you consume the plant-derived ALA, a small portion will be converted in your body to the fish oil compounds EPA and DHA. This makes it difficult to tell which of these compounds, the ALA or the EPA/DHA, is exerting a beneficial effect. As a result, the evidence for ALA is less compelling. That being said, there are multiple studies that suggest the regular consumption of ALA is good for your cardiovascular health. Specifically, it is thought to lessen your chances of having a heart attack, and also lower your blood pressure.[15,16]

One word of caution, though: If you have a history of prostate cancer, you might want to limit dietary intake of this substance as there is conflicting data about whether its intake may lead to a more aggressive form of this cancer.[17]

While the evidence for ALA is somewhat limited, the evidence for EPA and DHA, the fish oil compounds, is not. There is a mountain of studies demonstrating their effectiveness in multiple different disease states. While the evidence may be stronger for some disease states than for others, the overall impression is that fish oils are good for your health. The challenge is sifting through all the available data to find the most compelling reason to take these compounds.

In the arena of cardiovascular health, fish oils appear to be most effective. Their regular consumption has been found to reduce first heart attacks, repeat heart attacks, cardiovascular death, and overall mortality.[18,19,20]

The numbers may differ slightly from study to study, but the decrease in cardiovascular death is thought to be about 25 percent, and the decrease in overall mortality about 20 percent. Their intake has also been shown to lower your triglyceride levels by 20 to 50 percent, which may be one of the reasons why they are so beneficial to your heart.[21,22]

In regard to other conditions, there are a lot of disease states where fish-oil consumption may possibly be effective. The list includes such varied diseases as asthma, attention deficit disorder, dementia, depression, high blood pressure, psoriasis, rheumatoid arthritis, and strokes, to name just a few. The take-home point is that these seemingly unrelated diseases may all be potentially improved by the intake of fish oils. Further study is needed, but it is amazing to think that one substance may affect so many other conditions. These compounds appear to be safe, but they may slightly increase your risk of bleeding, so you should check with your doctor before using them. Otherwise, they are well-tolerated by most people.

As to the dose, the American Heart Association recommends an intake of 1 gram/day of the fish oils, EPA and DHA, or 1.5 to 3 grams/day of the plant-derived alpha linolenic acids, ALA, for adults with documented coronary artery disease. If you have never had a heart problem, it is recommended that you eat a variety of fish twice a week, and you are urged to use oils rich in ALA such as canola, flaxseed, and soybean oils. When you buy your fish, you should know that even fish cannot make their own omega-3 compounds. Rather, they acquire these oils by feeding off algae. As a result, there can be a significant difference in EPA and DHA levels between farmed and wild-caught salmon. The wild-caught salmon will have a lot more.

Not for All the Green Tea in China . . .

While the health benefits of fish oils were not discovered until the 1970s, the suspected health benefits of green tea date back a little further. The Chinese Emperor Shen Nung is credited with the discovery of tea and its mysterious healing powers roughly 5,000 years ago.

Known as China's Father of Medicine and Father of Agriculture, Emperor Shen Nung experimented with all different types of herbs, searching for ones with medicinal properties. As legend has it, a burning tea leaf inadvertently floated into his cup of water, yielding an enticing aroma. The Emperor then sipped this concoction of nature, making him the first person ever to taste a cup of tea. He started trying this plant as a remedy for many ailments, and quickly became impressed with its amazing ability to cure a whole host of conditions. From here, the legend of tea has only grown and grown.

Why would tea have healing properties? As you have seen with chocolate and wine, when certain foods and beverages are derived from plant sources, they may retain some of the plant's natural protective compounds. Polyphenols, as these substances are called, are designed to repair any damage done to the plant from the environment, serving as the plant's de facto first line of defense. When consumed by humans, they seem to possess similar healing properties by acting like very potent antioxidants. When it comes to tea, the challenge becomes extracting as much of the polyphenols from the tea leaf as possible to achieve the maximum health benefit.

The majority of tea comes from the leaves of a plant known as *Camellia sinensis,* which is found primarily in India, Japan, and China. Basically, there are three different types of tea that can be brewed from the leaves of this plant, depending on how quickly the leaves are steamed or heated after being harvested. When the leaves are heated immediately, you get green tea; when they are heated after thirty minutes, you get oolong tea; and when they are heated after sixty minutes, you get black tea. From the plant's perspective, when it is harvested, it is being injured. Therefore, it tries to heal itself by using the polyphenol compounds in its leaves. These polyphenols become activated when the integrity of the leaf is violated, as occurs with harvesting. By quickly steaming or heating the leaves, the chemical reaction that breaks down the polyphenols so they can be used is stopped in its tracks. Thus the sooner the leaves are heated, the sooner the chemical process is stopped, and the higher the polyphenol content in the tea will be. This is why green tea is thought to be healthiest. It has the highest polyphenol content, and the greatest antioxidant activity.

Over the years, clear preferences have evolved, with Western societies primarily choosing black tea and Eastern societies primarily choosing green tea. From these inclinations, epidemiologists have been looking for trends that would support the claim that green tea is healthier for you. One example often cited is the fact that Eastern countries in general, and Japan in particular, have a much lower incidence of both heart disease and lung cancer compared to their Western counterparts. This has been found, despite the fact that there is much higher tobacco consumption in the Eastern countries, a behavior which would be expected to increase, not decrease, both of these medical conditions. The *Asian paradox,* as this has been called, has made many wonder whether the high consumption of green tea is the explanation for this phenomenon.[23]

One problem with this type of speculation lies in the fact that it is difficult to prove causality. While the incidence of heart disease is lower in Japan and the consumption of green tea is high, it may be possible that the two, although true, may be unrelated. Another reasonable explanation could focus on the Japanese diet that is high in fish and the omega-3 fatty acids.

Like the little engine that could, green tea has slowly, but steadily, gained credibility over the years, as more and more studies have demonstrated its efficacy. These studies have primarily concentrated on green tea's ability to improve cardiovascular health and prevent cancer. Although limited, the studies of its impact on heart disease seem to suggest that consuming three to ten cups of green tea daily lowers your cholesterol, lowers your overall risk for having a heart attack, and lowers your risk of dying from any cause.[24,25,26]

With regard to cancer prevention, there is a lot of interest in green tea and excitement about its possible effectiveness. Studies have shown that it may lower your risk of developing many different types of cancer, including bladder cancer, esophageal cancer, ovarian cancer, and pancreatic cancer.[27,28,29]

There is conflicting data whether it may help with stomach and breast cancer, with some studies showing benefit, and others not.[30,31]

That being said, the general impression is that green tea exhibits some protective benefits when it comes to cancer, and given its relative safety, it has become the most common supplement used by American cancer patients.[32]

As with red wine and chocolate, flavonoids are also thought to be the compound affording all the health benefits in green tea. Researchers have been able to study its makeup, and they have isolated a particular flavonoid known as EGCG. (Its chemical name is epigallo-catechin-3-gallate, but even scientists refer to it as the abbreviated EGCG.) In your body, this compound is thought to act like a potent antioxidant, deactivating your bad cholesterol, and making it less likely to form plaque. As for cancer, tumor cells are dependent on the creation of new blood vessels in order to grow and survive. EGCG limits this growth of new blood vessels, effectively crippling tumor cells before they take hold and before they can spread.

If green tea has been around for 5,000 years, why is there only limited data on its effectiveness? Given that tea is the most consumed beverage on the planet, there was little incentive for the drug companies to study it. People were already consuming it in large amounts. But this is starting to change. With the discovery of EGCG, and with the realization that green tea may possess some anti-cancer properties, the health benefits of green tea are no longer being taken for granted.

The Natural Wonders of the World

When I was in high school, my biology teacher, Mr. Gallagher, would start off each semester by drawing a circle on the blackboard. The inside of the circle represents all your current knowledge, he would say, while the perimeter around the circle is the limits of what you know. As you learn, your circle gets bigger, since your knowledge base grows. He would draw a second, bigger circle on the blackboard to emphasize this point. He then would trace with his finger the larger perimeter of the second circle to show that, as your knowledge base grows, so too does the limit of your knowledge. This means that *the more you know, the more you know you don't know.*

Mr. Gallagher went through this exercise for several reasons. First, he was not trying to discourage his students, but rather to inspire us. He hoped to instill in us the same sense of wonder he possessed about the subject he had pursued his whole life. His basic premise is that science doesn't have to be boring. If you hang in there long enough, you will eventually come upon things that will intrigue you.

Second, he wanted to dispel the natural tendency of students to think we have already learned everything there is to know about a subject. The study of science doesn't work that way. It is a dynamic, ever-changing discipline that requires continual vigilance in its ultimate goal of discovering the truth.

Students are not the only ones who tend to be presumptuous. Teachers, researchers, and doctors also exhibit the same tendency to think they have learned everything there is to know about a subject. When something challenges the currently accepted truth by behaving in an unexpected way, the term *paradox* is used, implying there is a problem in the object being studied, rather than in the observer. Paradox is a friendlier way of saying there is a gap in our understanding, a friendlier way of saying we just don't know all there is to know.

So, a debt of gratitude is owed to the Kuna Indians of Central America, to the French along the Mediterranean coast, to the Inuits of Greenland, and to the Japanese of Asia for their help in enlightening the rest of us, and enlarging our circle. A debt of gratitude is also owed to the researchers studying these groups of people from around the world. It was their open-mindedness and willingness to challenge the status quo that allowed the rest of us to take a major step forward in our understanding. These cultures have shown that many different paths can be followed in the perpetual quest for healthier living.

Nature's Tips for Health

1. Alcohol in any form, when consumed in moderation, may actually be healthy for you. Limit yourself to one drink per day if you are female, or one to two drinks per day if you are male. WARNING: Be very careful. If you have a family history of alcoholism, avoid the temptation all together.

2. If you enjoy red wine, you should choose a full-bodied wine, such as a Pinot Noir or a Cabernet Sauvignon. By doing this, you should

receive additional health benefits from the polyphenols in the skin of the grape, above and beyond what you would receive from drinking alcohol alone.

3. Choose dark chocolate with the highest cocoa content to receive the greatest benefit. When consuming chocolate, watch the sugar and fats that are frequently added, as they will quickly nullify any of the health benefits inherent in the dark chocolate.

4. Omega-3 fatty acids come from both plants and fish. The fish-derived omega-3 compounds are known as EPA and DHA, and the data for their use is strong. Attempt to eat coldwater fish twice a week, or take 1 gram per day of these compounds.

5. If you have a hard time tolerating the omega-3 fish oils because of indigestion or the fishy burp, try freezing the capsules, then swallowing them. This usually eliminates the problem.

6. Green tea is the preferable type to drink, as it has a higher polyphenol content than other teas. Its use has been connected with improving your cardiovascular health and preventing cancer.

7. In the cultures studied, whether you are talking about the Kuna Indians of Central America, the French along the Mediterranean coast, the Inuit Eskimos of Greenland, or the Japanese of Asia, the amount of flavonoids and/or fish oils they consume on a daily basis is very high. To reach similar levels, you will likely have to take some form of a supplement. Given that these four active compounds are not typically found together, you should look for them on food and supplement labels.

   • Resveratrol (red wine)

   • Epicatechin (chocolate)

   • EPA and DHA (fish oils)

   • EGCG (green tea)

8

WAIST MANAGEMENT

Hunger is a sweet sauce.
—DAD HENNESSY

It may be that the taste of extra salty french fries is imprinted in the pleasure center of my brain. It may be that the convenience of eating food prepared by someone else is too hard to resist. Or, it may simply be that the advertising experts have been successful in their ability to manipulate my behavior. Whatever the reason, I have to admit that I love fast food. This fact, although somewhat embarrassing, is undeniable. Each and every time I reward myself with this treat, I get an exhilarating rush.

As soon as I turn into the parking lot, my heart rate speeds up, my mood lightens, and my mouth waters in anticipation of the feast that is about to come. Frankly, there is not much difference between my reaction and the reaction a dog conditioned to come running once the dinner bell is rung might exhibit. I am basically wagging my tail as I patiently wait for the worker to give me my food.

Over the years, I have developed fond memories of these visits to the fast food restaurants. While some people may remember how they felt when we first landed on the moon, I can still recall how I felt the first time I was introduced to the concept of *supersizing* my meal. When asked if I would like to double the size of my food order for a few extra cents, it only took a fraction of a second to come to the realization that this was a good thing—a very good thing. I remember that my knee-jerk response, "Hell yeah," drew attention from the other customers in the store that day because it had been a little too quick, a little too loud, and a little too enthusiastic. It would probably not have been my phrase of choice if I had actually *thought* about my response, but when dealing with the acquisition of food, a primal force ensuring survival sometimes takes hold of my brain. I can't imagine anyone actually saying no to the supersize question. In many ways, it seems analogous to the ATM machine asking whether I would like an extra ten dollar bill for the small surcharge of fifty cents. "Hell yeah" would be blurted out again.

Another memory I distinctly recall involved the first time I was introduced to the concept of *unlimited refills*. As the cashier had explained it to me, in an effort to save time, the restaurant was asking its customers to fill their own drinks. For this major inconvenience, she went on to say, I was entitled to drink as much as I wanted. Losing control to my primal force again, I strained my neck vigorously nodding my assent. It was easy to acknowledge this as a great idea— a classic *win-win* situation for both patron and business.

Before that day, I had never drunk 60 ounces of soda at one sitting, but that day I was drinking even though I wasn't thirsty. I was performing my own taste test, sampling all the available brands of beverage. I was even filling my cup as I left the store to ensure that I had gotten my money's worth. The caffeine headache that predictably followed had taken close to six hours to subside. Why this didn't serve as a deterrent for future ventures I can't really say, but it didn't.

One memory of which I am not too proud involves my discovery of the *bonus fries*. After a particularly gluttonous meal, when my hunger had been completely satisfied, I reached into the food bag and came across a few fries that had escaped from their container. Bonus fries, as they quickly got named, caused a definite thrill to go through my body. They became the perfect ending to the eating feast. Unfortunately, they also became the outward symbol of how low I could go, as they often made me feel like a starving person searching a trash can for food, even though, pathetically enough, I would be far from starving.

Fortunately, although I have not entirely shaken my mania for fast food, in my case I *am* able to limit my fast-food forays to once or twice a month. It seems that a number of people out there are fighting similar battles trying to resist the incredibly strong temptations of *bad* foods.

As this new century starts, it is painfully obvious that, collectively, the nation is losing more of these battles than it is winning. The statistics are not lying when they suggest that the majority of Americans are overweight. What amazes me, though, is despite all the time, money, and effort spent to combat this problem, this statistic is still true. Everyone desperately wants to be able to control their weight, and most people would do just about anything to achieve this goal. The problem arises in both knowing what to do and consistently doing it.

Generally, people have lost confidence in the popular diets, as they don't seem to work in the long run; they have lost confidence in the advice of experts on what to eat, for they don't really seem to know; and they have lost confidence in their own ability to change behavior because they've proven to themselves that they can't. I believe the secret to regaining this lost confidence lies in a better understanding of why people behave the way they do, and that, once equipped with this knowledge, they will be much better prepared to make the changes necessary for ultimate success.

A High Price to Pay—Obesity's Impact on Society

The problem of obesity—both its wide scope and its strong contribution to so many medical conditions—is arguably the greatest health threat facing the United States. Statistics show that 64.5 percent of adult Americans are overweight, 30 percent of these are obese, and close to 5 percent are extremely obese. And, when talking about young Americans, the numbers are downright discouraging, as 13 percent of all children are also considered overweight.[1,2]

Alarmingly, these numbers are only getting worse. Since 1980, the percentage of obese Americans has doubled, and the percentage of overweight children has tripled. Reviewing these numbers, most experts quite accurately describe the situation as an epidemic that is unprecedented in United States history.

What the consequences will be is a frightening notion to entertain, and a difficult one to predict. As excessive weight contributes to a whole array of conditions, there will clearly be medical fallout from this epidemic. It is well known that obesity contributes to higher rates of heart disease, higher blood-pressure readings, and higher cholesterol numbers. As a result, there will be an increased number of overweight people taking more medications to combat these conditions. It is also widely accepted that obesity is the primary cause of type 2 diabetes which, in itself, has its own links to many medical problems. Obesity is known to increase the risk of breast, colon, and endometrial cancers. It is known to increase the risk for arthritis, with knees being especially vulnerable, and it often is associated with chronic back pains.

Obesity is perhaps most damaging psychologically, as low self-esteem and depression are frequent cohabiters with this condition. Underscoring this point, one study of previously obese people who underwent successful gastric bypass surgery found that 100 percent of them would prefer being deaf, 91.5 percent would prefer having a leg amputated, and 89.4 percent would prefer being blind to being obese again.[3]

The economic fallout from obesity is equally staggering. It is estimated that the United States is now spending somewhere between 75 billion and 100 billion dollars a year on weight-related diseases. And the American public is currently spending another $33 billion on the commercial diet industry in a desperate effort not to be heavy.[4]

Lost productivity from missed workdays, lost wages from medical illness, and lost opportunity from underemployment are all variables that are difficult to measure accurately, but nevertheless need to be factored into the overall equation. This increased spending on weight-related problems eventually gets passed down to the small business owners and individual consumers who are forced to pay higher insurance premiums for healthcare. In both dollars spent and life years lost, there will be an increasing price to pay for this epidemic.

A logical question is, if billions of dollars are being spent on the obesity problem, then why is it so difficult for so many people to lose weight? It would seem that weight management is not quite as simple as some of the clichés would have it. Although *eat less, exercise more* serves as a good sound bite, it lacks insight into the more complex processes that actually determine a person's weight. These processes are governed by an interplay between biological, behavioral, environmental, and dietary forces that affect different people in different ways. For some, biology may be the strongest contributor to the weight problem. For others, behavioral and dietary factors may prevail. So, in order to best manage them, it is crucial to have an understanding of how much, and in what areas, these forces are exerting their influence.

BIOLOGICAL FORCES

Excessive Energy Storage—Too Much of a Good Thing

Energy must be acquired, stored, and reused if a living being is expected to do anything. The human body attempts to adhere to this natural law by acquiring its energy through the intake of food, by storing it in the form of fat cells, and by reusing it through a complex series of reactions that essentially transform oxygen and sugar into functional energy units. The proper functioning of this energy network is critical to the long-term survival of the species. As a result, by the Darwinian law of natural selection, the body has evolved a fairly sophisticated digestive system, one in which the various parts are able to communicate with each other through the use of chemical messengers. It is these chemical messengers that are primarily responsible for individuals behaving as they do. For example, they exert control over appetite and cravings, they affect meal initiation and termination, and they regulate the body's overall rate of energy expenditure. Through these actions, the body is able to match energy intake with energy output. In an ideal setting, these numbers should be about equal.

By most scientific standards, the body serves as a highly efficient power plant. The average person consumes close to a million calories during a given year, yet usually keeps weight gain to within a five-pound margin. The problem, of course, is that over time those five pounds start adding up.

It may be helpful to visualize the interactions taking place by thinking of the digestive system as a symphony orchestra. The various organs, such as the gallbladder, pancreas, and stomach, all have a part to play, which they do while trying to simultaneously harmonize with each other. This synchronicity is accomplished by the exchange of the chemical messengers that travel throughout the system. These messengers elicit responses from the different organs, either increasing their activity or shutting them down. The brain, the de facto conductor, is ultimately in charge. Its messengers supersede all others, and it is continually listening to the messages being sent by the different parts of the system. The end result is that the *music* being made by the digestive system affects the brain—and by extension, the body—and causes it to behave in certain ways. It is the very complexity of this system itself, with its built-in protection against rapid weight loss, that, in many ways, prevents weight-management plans from being successful.

The Hunger Hormone that Drives Appetite

Ghrelin, one of the most interesting chemical messengers, was discovered in 1999. Produced in the stomach and nicknamed the hunger hormone, its discovery is thought to potentially be a major breakthrough for obesity treatment. Prior to the three main meals a day that most people eat, ghrelin's level has been consistently found to be elevated, implying that it has a definite role in making people eat. In addition to increasing food intake, it appears that ghrelin "affects all aspects of the energy-regulation system in a concerted manner to promote weight gain."[5]

Some experts believe that ghrelin is the major culprit underlying the yo-yo diet, a dieting pattern familiar to nearly everyone who has ever tried to lose weight. Initial weight loss, followed by an almost compensatory higher weight gain, has made more than one expert wonder whether most people would be better off never dieting in the first place. Studies have shown that individuals who have lost as little as 5 percent of their body weight have marked elevations of circulating ghrelin levels lasting months.[6]

The increased ghrelin levels are thought to be directly related to regaining weight because, unfortunately, any diet that causes rapid weight loss will likely have a corresponding rise in this hormone. Interestingly, some researchers are proposing that the long-term success of gastric bypass surgery is more dependent on inhibiting the secretions of this hormone than on limiting the size of the stomach cavity.

The Appetite-Suppressing Hormone

Ghrelin, the only known appetite stimulant, is counterbalanced by several hormones produced largely in the small intestine that function as appetite suppressants. Peptide YY, commonly abbreviated as PYY, and glucagon-like peptide-1, abbreviated as GLP-1, are probably the best known of these hormones. PYY became popular in September 2003 when an article in the *New England Journal of Medicine* reported that obese individuals had demonstrated lower levels of PYY in their system when compared to normal controls. When the same obese individuals received an infusion of PYY, their caloric intake decreased by an incredible 30 percent. It was immediately speculated that a deficiency of this hormone could be a major player in the development of obesity. GLP-1 also gained popularity in September 2003 when an article in the *Journal of Nutrition* reported that the dietary intake of protein lessens appetite by stimulating the GLP-1 pathway.[7,8]

For years, the disciples of the low-carbohydrate approach to dieting have claimed to be less hungry. This, in part, may be validated by the actions of GLP-1. The discovery of these naturally occurring appetite suppressants has provided an excellent opportunity for the drug companies to develop products that might mimic their activity. Safe, well-tolerated, and effective appetite suppressants could revolutionize the weight-loss industry. Their discovery has also provided an explanation as to why some people reach the sensation of fullness faster than others. By better understanding these appetite-suppressant signals, it is hoped that doctors will be better able to counsel people in their efforts to lose weight.

A Failure to Communicate

The discovery of leptin in 1994 represented a major breakthrough in uncovering the biology underlying weight control. Prior to that date, most researchers viewed fat as a passive, metabolically silent storage unit, lacking any ability to interact with its surroundings. It is now known that your fat cells can make their own chemical messenger, leptin, that can signal the brain about the extent of its energy storage. Increased fat stores lead to higher levels of leptin, which tell your brain to decrease food intake and increase energy expenditure. Given the current epidemic of obesity, it is becoming obvious for all to see that this hormone has *not* been successful in doing its job.[9]

There are literally dozens of these chemical messengers. It is not important to try to learn them all. Rather, it is important to know they exist. Your body has evolved a highly complex system to store energy. As might be expected with any complex system, there are multiple places where something might not work properly. This may help to explain why certain weight-loss approaches may work better for some people than for others. Some may not be able to increase their internal energy expenditure, so a diet focusing on calorie restriction would work best for them. Others may have a low level of PYY in their system, so they might do better on a high-protein diet in order to suppress their appetite through the GLP-1 system. This concept would also help explain how genetics may be involved. It is very possible that people may inherit deficiencies in one or more of the chemical messengers, thus predisposing them to be overweight.

It is widely accepted that your body tries to maintain balance in its energy-storage system. When people intentionally try to lose weight, they are upsetting this balance. As a result, compensatory reactions will take place to restore the norm and regain the weight. Similar compensatory reactions are supposed to be triggered to offset weight gain. Unfortunately, this system gets frequently overwhelmed by the excessive caloric intake currently seen in society. Through changes in the food industry, most of them aimed at increased profits rather than any increased well-being of customers, this excessive intake has been made easier and easier.

ENVIRONMENTAL FORCES

Living in a High-Calorie World

Throughout the last century, Americans as a whole gradually became heavier. Attributable to the abundant food supply, the relative prosperity of America, and a less physically active lifestyle, this weight gain should not have been unexpected.

In the 1970s everything seemed to change. The rate at which people gained weight began increasing significantly. Many theories were put forth to try to explain this phenomenon, with most focusing on changes taking place in the food industry. My own personal experiences noted at the beginning of this chapter illustrate this development. Almost simultaneously, food preparation changed with the creation of a cheaper processed sugar, food delivery changed with the appearance of larger portion sizes, and food marketing changed with the development of high-budget advertising campaigns. All these watershed changes occurred when the majority of households started having two people in the work force. This shift in society left much less time and energy for food preparation, a fact the food industry intentionally exploited. The biologic forces described above were designed primarily to protect against rapid weight loss when food was scarce, and they were ill-equipped to handle the mass influx of high-calorie foods that occurred when food was abundant.

Great Taste, Less Filling—How HFCS Promotes Weight Gain

In the late 1970s, the origins of the obesity epidemic began to take hold about the time a new sweetener, high-fructose corn syrup (HFCS), started appearing on food labels. It didn't take long for many experts to speculate this could be more than just a coincidence. This inexpensive sugar, which replaced cane sugar as the preferred sweetener of the food industry, can now be found in nearly everything. The major question being asked by researchers is whether it is to blame for the fattening of America.

Most experts in the field of obesity agree that HFCS must bear some responsibility for enabling food makers to sell products in larger portions. The food industry quickly realized that great profits could be made by enriching and enlarging products with this cheap sugar. A major debate remains, though, as to whether the fructose in this sweetener is more fattening than its predecessors. Some argue that fructose is metabolized differently than other sugars. They believe it is much more easily converted into fat, and is a much weaker appetite suppressant. They go on to argue that people don't get the signal to stop eating when they eat foods high in HFCS and, as a result, they eat a lot more. More research is needed to investigate these claims, and on this compound, in general, given that it is consumed in such large quantities by nearly all Americans.

Giving the World a Coke

In becoming the most popular sweetener, high-fructose corn syrup has had its greatest impact on the soda industry. Reflected primarily in serving sizes, high-fructose corn syrup was instrumental in the conversion from the 12 ounce can of the 1970s to the 20 ounce bottle of the 1990s. As could be expected with such a change, soda consumption, particularly among adolescents, rose sharply. One study analyzing this trend demonstrated a 300 percent increase in the amount of soda consumed in America during this time period. No wonder obesity rates started to rise around this same time. The problem with excessive calorie intake through soda is that it tends to add to, but not displace, calories taken in by other dietary measures.[10,11]

When you consider that the typical 20 ounce bottle of soda contains the equivalent of fourteen teaspoons of sugar and close to 300 calories of energy, it is easy to understand how difficult it is to offset that intake by burning more calories through increased physical activity. Most people can't do it, and they are getting fatter as a result.

In an effort to balance their budgets, in the 1990s, school districts began entering into exclusive *pouring-rights* contracts with soda companies. In the beginning, it would have been difficult to argue with the reasoning of school administrators. The vending machines were already in the school cafeterias, the students were already drinking soda on a regular basis, and the money being offered was really needed to help keep the schools fiscally sound. Unfortunately, things did not work out as planned. These pouring-rights contracts were often incentive-based, rewarding schools for selling more soda to students. Schools often allowed fairly liberal advertising on their grounds, and the unintended effect of these business arrangements was the not-so-subtle encouragement for students to consume not less, but more, soda.

Many health professionals rightly felt the school districts were selling out, sacrificing the health of their students to save some money. Given the public outcry, schools became less likely to consider these business arrangements, but as recently as the start of the 2002–2003 school year, there were still over 240 school districts honoring these contracts.[12,13] It became obvious that school officials needed some help.

As a result, the Alliance for a Healthier Generation was born. This is a joint initiative between the American Heart Association and the William J. Clinton Foundation. Their goal is to provide students with a healthier range of choices when it comes to beverages. Together with the American Beverage Association, they developed national guidelines that mandated that lower-calorie, more nutritious drinks be available to children in their schools. Thus far, their efforts have been overwhelmingly successful. The next challenge, it would seem, would be applying these standards to the home environment.

The Bigger, the Better?

The trend toward larger serving sizes was not unique to the soft drink industry, however. It reflected a broader pattern of increased portion sizes throughout all aspects of the food industry that began in the 1970s and accelerated in the 1980s. A study published in the *American Journal of Public Health* in February 2002 documented rather dramatically the extent of this phenomenon. It showed that, by the 1990s, common foods, such as cookies, muffins, and pasta, had increased in serving size by an incredible 300 to 700 percent.[14]

A similar study, published by the *Journal of the American Medical Association* in January 2003, showed that the portion sizes and caloric intake for all key foods (except pizza) in the United States had increased substantially from 1977 to 1996.[15]

American waistlines showed a growth rate that paralleled this increase, which seems to indicate that when people are presented with larger quantities of food, they will eat more. And statistically, the data appear to support this claim. In the mid-1990s, Americans consumed 200 calories more every day than did their counterparts in the mid-1970s, largely due to the environmental forces that provided the public with abundant quantities of inexpensive, calorie-packed foods. Factor into this equation the well-funded marketing juggernaut aimed at influencing people's behavior—encouraging them to eat more—and the causes underlying the obesity epidemic begin to come into focus.[16]

BEHAVIORAL FORCES

Empty Calories—Eating Without Hunger

In terms of their contribution to obesity, the relationship between behavioral and environmental forces might be best explained by the old adage: *You can lead a horse to water, but you can't make him drink.* Late in the last century and continuing into this one, the environment has provided the horse with plenty of water to drink, but ultimately it is always up to the horse to determine how much it will drink. By making an abundant food supply readily available, some people, perhaps due to their biologic makeup, find it easy to control their eating behavior, and as a result, are able to limit their overall intake. Others are not so lucky.

Eating behaviors can be broken down into those involved with meal initiation, those involved with the eating of the meal, and those involved with meal termination. Problems in any of these three areas may lead to a person becoming overweight.

Meal initiation, when triggered by hunger, is normal and healthy. It is when it is triggered for reasons other than hunger that it becomes problematic. Obviously, there are many reasons why people eat when they're not hungry, with anxiety, depression, and heightened stress being particularly common. In these instances, people are not eating for sustenance, but rather for comfort. The act of eating makes them feel good. The mere sight or smell of food often invokes pleasurable responses and propels them to action. When people gather in groups, there is also a tendency to begin eating, even though there may be no hunger. These situations frequently result in opportunistic eating, just because the food is there; nervous eating because they don't know what to say; and bored eating because they don't know what to do.

Home Cooking—Where Have You Gone?

Where people choose to eat also influences how much they will eat. In the 1970s, food consumed outside the home accounted for approximately 35 percent of the family's food budget. In the 1990s and early 2000s, this number came closer to 45 to 50 percent.[17,18]

With the well-documented larger portion sizes found throughout the food industry, this trend clearly impacted on the likelihood of people becoming overweight. It is now obvious that people are eating less and less of the three major meals at home, leading to the natural conclusion that this will only add to the number of overweight individuals in the future.

The impact attributed to eating out may be partially blunted, however, because behaviors at home also appear to be changing, and not for the better. Perhaps influenced by the bigger meals they have been receiving when they eat out, people are choosing to prepare much larger portion sizes at home. This seems to reflect the gradual development of increased expectations that more food should be prepared and eaten in order to satisfy needs. This change represents a different mindset with ramifications that can be far-reaching.[19]

The trend toward larger portion sizes is particularly problematic as most people tend to clean their plates, finishing all the food that is put in front of them. Overeating results when people fail to recognize they have consumed enough. This inability to control behavior and terminate meals when hunger is satisfied is one of the primary causes underlying the obesity epidemic. The phenomenon is most noticeable when people are distracted, as when they are watching television, talking with others, or attending movies. When there is no conscious thought telling them to stop what they are doing, people will mindlessly keep eating, often consuming incredible amounts of food without ever appreciating that they had done so.

In general, it seems that people are expecting to eat more; their biologic systems are adapting to eat more; environmental changes are helping them eat more; and behaviors are adjusting to eat more. It is in this context that the makeup of a diet should be examined.

DIETARY FORCES

The Great Debate—Calories vs. Carbohydrates

Traditionally, a person's diet gets the most attention as the reason why he or she may be heavy. This is the most analyzed, most discussed, most debated, and least understood aspect of the obesity epidemic. Researchers have analyzed the diets of people in almost every way imaginable, yet they still cannot come to an agreement as to what would be considered good to eat. The foods that people consume can be described by their energy content (i.e., how many calories are present); by their macronutrient contents (i.e., how many carbohydrates, proteins, and fats are present); and by the extent to which they have been processed (i.e., made into too-rapidly assimilated energy sources). Except for processed foods, each type has its own cheerleaders as to what represents the perfect diet. Some concentrate solely on the energy content of food by having people count calories, while others focus more on the specific amounts of carbohydrates or fats. It is not important to understand every aspect of the many diets on the market. Rather, it will be much more productive for you to appreciate some of the major principles on which these diets are based. In this manner, you can take suggestions from the different strategies, and create a diet that best meets your particular likes and dislikes.

Counting Calories

For many, it is all about the calories. "A calorie is a calorie is a calorie" is the oft-quoted tenet of the philosophy that weight gain will predictably follow when calorie consumption exceeds calorie expenditure. This expenditure is the sum total of energy that the body needs to run itself. Even at rest, the body is continually burning calories to run its thousands of internal reactions. When the extra calories to power the body's physical activity are factored into the equation, a definite number, expressed in total calories expended, can be calculated. This number can then be compared to the total calories of the food consumed to see whether you will be gradually gaining or losing weight over time. Theoretically, through a combination of decreased intake and increased expenditure, you would have to account for 3,500 calories to lose one pound of weight.

The advantages to this type of approach are primarily gained by those taking personal responsibility for their actions. Eat less and exercise more can be easily traced back to this philosophy. It encourages you to watch your portion sizes, and it encourages you to be more physically active.

By counting the calories in the food you eat, you can once again take control of your weight, or so the theory goes. But, there are a few pitfalls with this strategy. Although relatively easy to comprehend, it can be tedious to put into practice. It takes a considerable amount of time and effort to count calories consistently. When a lack of immediate results is added to these pressures, it is easy to see why many can get frustrated and start looking elsewhere for answers to their weight problems.

A deeper concern is whether weight control is all about the calories. On the surface, it would seem undeniable that caloric mismatch is at the core of the weight-management problem. Upon closer inspection, though, the numbers don't always seem to add up. Some people are unable to lose weight despite Herculean efforts to limit calories, while others lose more than their halfhearted effort rightfully deserves.

One theory, which may partially explain this phenomenon, is that if you intentionally restrict the intake of your calories, you create an artificial environment that fools your body into thinking a food shortage might be present. In this instance, built-in mechanisms designed to ensure survival will likely be enacted to limit the rate at which your body burns calories. By decreasing its basal metabolic rate, your body will, in essence, be minimizing the impact that the self-imposed, restricted-calorie intake might bring.

Another concern with the all-about-calories approach is whether people are able to correctly measure intake or expenditure of calories in the first place. All foods carry a potential caloric load. Whether this caloric load actually gets realized may depend on several factors. How fast the food moves through your digestive system, how much energy your body needs at any given moment, and how the calories are packaged in terms of carbohydrates, fats, and proteins may all impact on how much of the calorie content you ultimately absorb.

This may help to explain why some people can seemingly eat and eat without ever gaining any weight, while others gain weight simply by looking at food. If it were only about calories, then both groups, the chronically thin and the chronically fat, with approximately the same activity level, should gain and lose weight at the same rate, based on what they eat. And this clearly doesn't happen.

On the expenditure side, a calorie, much like a dollar amount, can certainly be applied to any physical activity. A thirty-minute walk, for example, might cost your body 200 calories. The assumption, though, is that your body will only have to spend that amount. The actual cost may depend on whether or not the calories are readily available. Available calories, those circulating in your bloodstream in the form of sugar, can be used directly to pay the cost of any given activity. Unavailable calories, those in fat storage, must be retrieved first before they can be utilized. It is possible that this retrieval process may somehow throw off the calorie counts. Thus, the metabolic punch that exercise might bring may be very dependent on whether calories are available or not, and this, in turn, may be dependent on the timing of your last meal. Conceivably, the same exercise routine can yield very different results, depending on when it is done during the day.

Obviously, more research is needed to answer some of these questions. Counting calories may not be the only answer when it comes to weight management, but it is part of the answer, and its value should not be underestimated. Other factors, though, should also be considered when considering the weight control equation.

Counting Carbohydrates and Fats

Besides its calorie amount, does the composition of food, with regard to its carbohydrate, fat, and protein content, affect weight? This has proven to be a very difficult question to answer. Surprisingly, the merits of most diets have been based on their ability to decrease heart attacks, lessen plaque formation, and improve cholesterol numbers. Their ability to actually promote weight loss was almost forgotten in the studies—often unmentioned and rarely highlighted. As a result, evidence supporting any diet's claim of long-term weight control has been seriously lacking. Another problem is that experts frequently analyze diets using different sets of criteria. As an example, when comparing a low-fat diet to a low-carbohydrate diet, it is sometimes difficult to discern which set of criteria an expert might be using. To some, saying a diet is no good may mean it will likely contribute to higher rates of heart attacks and should not be followed. To others, this same expression may be interpreted as meaning the diet will not likely result in weight loss. The true meaning may get lost in the shuffle. These apples to oranges, decreasing heart attacks to decreasing weight comparisons, have greatly contributed to the confusion surrounding the dieting question, making it difficult for the average person to decide what is ultimately good to eat.

In America, in the latter half of the last century, the low-fat diet became the diet most recommended by health professionals, primarily because of its perceived ability to decrease heart attacks. Modeled chiefly after the Mediterranean diet, this type of diet generally recommends limiting fat to less than 30 percent of total daily intake, with special attention to limiting saturated fat to less than 10 percent. There have been numerous studies supporting the claim of fewer events (i.e., heart attacks) in people who follow this type of diet.[20,21,22,23]

Based on these studies, the American Heart Association, the federally funded Dietary Guidelines for Americans (a comprehensive report released every five years), and the Food Guide Pyramid have all adopted the general principle of limiting fat intake. The question remains, though, whether a diet low in fat promotes weight loss. This is a difficult question to answer for several reasons. Although there are studies demonstrating weight loss with the low-fat diets, there are usually other variables, such as restricted calorie intake, that may also be playing a role, but there are not many long-term studies looking into the matter. Ethically, researchers were reluctant to develop studies involving control groups with higher fat intake for fear they might be exposing the participants to higher risks of heart problems. As a result of this lack of study, most healthcare professionals combined the low-fat and low-calorie diets into one in order to achieve the benefits of decreased heart disease while simultaneously promoting weight loss.

The advantages of the union between low-fat and low-calorie diets are well known. Promoting individual responsibility, limiting portion sizes, and eating nutritiously all contribute to a healthy lifestyle, or so it is argued. The disadvantages of delayed results, poor long-term adherence, and lack of enjoyment, though, have also become all too familiar.

A major challenge was brought to the table by Dr. Robert Atkins in the 1980s when he noticed that the obesity epidemic seemed to coincide with the push toward low-fat diets (or high-carbohydrate as he would describe them). He argued it was the high consumption of carbohydrates that was driving the fattening of America.[24]

Through his efforts, and others like him, the low-carbohydrate craze dominated American culture throughout the 1990s and into the 2000s. Driven primarily by frustration from lack of results with the traditional diets, more people began turning to counting carbohydrates rather than counting calories as the last century came to a close. Carbohydrate diets became popular for several reasons. For many, they seemed to work when other diets hadn't. They also brought the enjoyment back to eating. By reintroducing previously banned foods, such as red meat and eggs, they helped to lift the cloud of boredom from most people's kitchens.

The question remains, "Do they work?" "Maybe," though not an attractive answer, is probably an accurate one. After reviewing all the studies performed prior to 2003 (about a hundred since the 1960s), researchers found there was "insufficient evidence" to recommend for or against these diets.[25]

The majority of these studies were limited to three months, and their designs were so variable that few solid conclusions could be drawn from their review. In latter stages of 2002 and the early part of 2003, there were three small studies, all six months in duration, in which people following low-carbohydrate diets demonstrated greater weight loss.[26,27,28]

Again, the design of the studies raised questions as to whether the carbohydrate composition was the sole variable that accounted for the observed weight loss. Despite this lack of scientific evidence, it was hard for physicians to ignore anecdotal reports of successful weight loss that kept getting reported by their patients. Detractors claim that much of this apparent success was from excessive fluid loss that is common in the early phases of these diets. They go on to argue that if long-term weight loss does occur, it results primarily from calorie restriction (i.e., people eating less), rather than from the carbohydrate composition of the food they eat.[29]

It is undeniable, though, that the low-carbohydrate philosophy has made major inroads into nutritional thinking. Even the most ardent disciples of the low-fat diets have started warning about the dangers of consuming too many of the *simple* carbohydrates. And a number of people have started to argue that the Food Pyramid should be revised to better highlight the fact that *all carbohydrates are not created equal.* Although scientifically there may be some doubt, there is no question in the minds of the pro-carbohydrate people as the pendulum of public opinion has swung in recent years to the low-carbohydrate craze. The debate is far from over. More long-term research is needed to better define what constitutes a healthy diet. Some have suggested that the extent of food processing should also be considered as it can *greatly* affect the amount of weight gained.

Counting Fiber

It might be most accurate to say that all foods carry a potential energy value. The challenge to your body is to absorb as much of this energy value as soon as possible. This task becomes more difficult when foods are closer to their natural state and contain higher amounts of fiber, fat, and protein, which slows absorption. When foods are processed, many of these elements have been stripped away, and once these natural, needed obstacles to slowed absorption are removed, the delicate balance of the digestive system gets thrown off, and a too-rapid absorption of energy usually results. This is usually manifested by a sudden elevation in blood sugar. When this happens, your body can either use the sugar to power one of its internal reactions, or more likely, convert it to fat for future use. Food processing, then, is responsible for presenting to your body a dysfunctional fuel, one stripped of all its natural protective components, and one destined to cause you many problems. Dr. Arthur Agatston, author of *The South Beach Diet*, best describes this situation when he explains that the faster sugars get absorbed in the body, the faster people tend to put on fat.[30]

Increasing fiber intake is probably the most helpful way to slow this absorption of food and blunt the energy surge that typically is seen. Unfortunately, for now, fiber is the Rodney Dangerfield of the food subclasses—it doesn't get any respect, though that is changing because fiber's benefits are hard to ignore. By regulating bowel movements, lowering cholesterol, hastening satiety, and delaying absorption, fiber can go a long way in helping to reach the goal of eventual weight control.

Finding the Healthy Diet for You

Over the years, I, like most people, have come to appreciate that long-term weight management is a very difficult thing to do. While invoking temporary changes is simple, sustainability is the real problem. The fast-paced world has everyone eating on the run, drinking excessive soda for the caffeine lift, and turning to food for comfort as much sustenance. So, despite all the good intentions, the weight-loss train frequently gets derailed.

What is a healthy diet? The answer really depends on who's asking the question. Personal likes and dislikes, genetics, eating behaviors, and environmental conditions all must be factored into the equation. What may be good for one person may not necessarily be right for the next. The major problem with diets in general is that they fail to recognize the true complexity of the body where many variables need to be considered if long-term weight loss is to be achieved.

Weight Loss Tips

1. Biological. Never skip meals. If meals are skipped, your body will release hunger hormones in an effort to ensure self-preservation. As

a result, bad food choices will be much more likely to happen because these hormones are practically impossible to resist.

2. Biological. Avoid the *winter-coat* syndrome. If you charted your weight throughout the year, you, like most people, would maintain a fairly stable weight because your body is highly efficient at matching energy intake with energy expenditure. Each winter, though, especially in northern climates, there tends to be a five-pound weight gain—the winter coat. For many reasons, it is extremely difficult not to gain this weight, and the problem arises when you don't remove the coat after the winter. If this happens, in just a few short years your weight can jump almost fifteen pounds. Since it's much easier to lose five pounds than fifteen pounds, each spring try to discipline yourself to get back to your pre-winter weight.

3. Environmental. Avoid foods that contain high-fructose corn syrup (HFCS), especially sodas and juices. It is important for parents to take a proactive role in limiting the soda intake of their children. Soda consumption, in record amounts, is one of the major contributors to adolescent obesity. Obese children almost always grow up to be obese adults. Help get the soda machines out of the schools, and you will be helping the health of your children.

4. Environmental. Be aware of portion sizes. The trend toward larger portion sizes, both at home and in restaurants, mirrors the trend of increasing weight. Read labels, check calories, and think about the amount of food you are consuming.

5. Behavioral. Weigh yourself weekly, and reward yourself with planned breaks.

6. Dietary forces. Limit foods that have high amounts of simple refined carbohydrates, saturated fats, and calories. *And, don't forget about increasing your fiber intake. Give it some respect.*

7. Behavioral. It is much better to be fit than to be thin. Most people get transfixed by the number on the scale rather than by their fitness level. When you build up your body, you will be building up your self-image, and isn't that why most people care about their weight in the first place?

9

SLEEP

*Early to bed, early to rise, makes a man healthy,
wealthy, and wise.*
—POOR RICHARD'S ALMANAC (EIGHTEENTH CENTURY)

*Late to bed, early to rise, makes a man tired,
caffeine-wired, and unwise.*
—POOR TIMOTHY'S ALMANAC (TWENTY-FIRST CENTURY)

In the fall of 1995, in the midst of my medical training, I learned the art of juggling, figuratively and literally. Newly married, working excessively long hours, and having limited time to pursue self-interests, I was forced to prioritize my time. Given that there was never enough time during the day to adequately meet these different needs, like most people, I began borrowing from the night. It would be nice to think this borrowing time from sleep was necessary to accomplish something important or achieve some higher good, but being in front of the TV, mindlessly changing channels, for example, falls far short of this lofty aim. Personal time, even when it involves doing nothing at all, is so coveted that many will sacrifice almost anything, especially sleep, to get it. Despite all the time-saving advances of technology, the great paradox of today is that people seem to have *less* rather than more personal time. As a result, they are forced to *rob Peter to pay Paul* by dipping into their sleep time in order to maintain adequate levels of personal time.

But this backfires because, without enough sleep, the tiredness perpetuates throughout the day, leading to your being less efficient at work, less fun to be around at home, and less fulfilled in your pursuit of self-interests—in essence, less likely to be happy. Some argue that this happiness is dependent on finding the right balance among the different spheres of life.

During one of my overnight calls, this concept of balance became crystal clear to me. Returning to my call room after working nineteen straight hours, I found a set of juggling balls on the nightstand. Obviously, at 2:00 AM the smart thing would be to grab some sleep if for no other reason than to be able to function the next day. The not-so-smart thing would be to start teaching myself how to juggle. Needless to say, I began tossing those balls into the air. Despite having fairly good hand-eye coordination, juggling was much more difficult than I anticipated. If I focused too much attention on any one ball, then I would drop them all. I also noticed, as I continued to practice, that I dropped the balls more frequently when I became more fatigued and less able to concentrate.

Somewhere in the middle of frequently dropping those balls, I became enlightened. I realized that, when sleep deprivation is mild, it tends to make people irritable; when it is extreme, however, sleep deprivation tends to make people high. In this context, I started becoming philosophical about my life, its purpose, and why I might be juggling balls in the early hours of the morning. Those balls started to become a metaphor for my life.

As I was desperately trying to find a balance among the competing demands of work, family, and self, I began seeing myself as that juggler, and seeing that when I didn't pay equal attention to these different facets of my life, I started having difficulty keeping those balls in the air. More than anything, it was this imbalance that caused me to feel stressed. I started noticing how stress would negatively affect my sleep. It was harder to fall asleep, harder to stay asleep, and harder to feel refreshed in the morning. This, coupled with the fact that I was voluntarily restricting my total sleep time so I could do important things, like juggle balls, created a situation wherein I was always tired—and a tired juggler is a bad juggler. My work suffered, my family life suffered, and my self-interests suffered.

Only when I made the conscious decision to sleep more did I begin to notice a difference—a *big* difference. I became more efficient at work, which allowed me to routinely get home sooner. I became happier, which improved the quality of my family time. And, with some creativity, I became better at finding some personal time too.

The key was applying value to sleep. *Time-management during the day was dependent on proper time-management during the night.*

Tiredness—Normal or Abnormal?

The sensation of feeling tired is so pervasive in society that most times it's not even considered abnormal, but rather a natural byproduct of living in today's fast-paced, competitive society. In most cases, this tiredness is dealt with by turning to ever increasing amounts of caffeine in coffees, teas, and sodas, literally getting a *fix* at the local coffee or donut shop to satisfy the addiction to artificial stimulants. Only when the tiredness gets to be excessive do people come into the office to see what may be wrong. And when I talk to them about their lack of sleep being the root cause of the problem, they become incredulous and find it hard to believe the answer could be that simple.

Why I Lay Me Down to Sleep

In many ways, sleep remains one of the great mysteries of life. Existence is literally dependent upon getting enough of it. Yet, amazingly, researchers do not fully understand why it is so important. In fact, it is humbling to think just how little is known about sleep, given that it consumes one-third of people's time on earth. It was only during the last seventy years or so that scientists even started to study sleep, often creating more questions than answers. It was always assumed that sleep was simply a passive process wherein the body and brain got needed time to recharge.

This concept began to be seriously challenged with the advent of the electroencephalograph (EEG). In 1930, Dr. Hans Berger, a German psychiatrist, noticed that electrical activity, and by extension, brain activity, could be measured by applying electrodes to the scalp. Almost immediately, this instrument showed there were differences between brain activity while awake and brain activity while asleep. The *alpha waves* of the awake brain disappeared completely when the person fell asleep, and this cessation of alpha-wave activity immediately became the gold standard by which scientists marked the beginning of sleep.[1]

In the 1930s and 40s, researchers developed a true appreciation for the complexity of sleep. Through the use of overnight EEGs, they were (rather unexpectedly) able to demonstrate that a typical night's sleep was composed of a wide assortment of brainwave activity. They noted periods of slow brainwave activity consistent with the idea that sleep was a passive time for recharging. But, they also noticed periods of heightened brainwave activity, at times more active than the awake brain, which they had a very difficult time explaining. In the 1950s, researchers Kleitman and Aserinsky discovered that this heightened brain activity was associated with jerky eye movements.[2]

This discovery of REM (*rapid eye movement*) sleep was a milestone in sleep research. It began the transition from thinking of sleep as a simple, passive process to understanding that it was much more complex, and this realization marked the beginning of contemporary sleep theory.

The Sleep Cycle

Most researchers believe the brain follows a natural progression when it sleeps. Usually within minutes of lying down, it eases into stage I—light sleep. It then is followed in rapid succession by sleep stages II, III, and IV, which correspond to deeper and deeper states of unconsciousness. Following stage IV sleep, the brain enters stage V, which is the Freudian world of REM sleep. It is a period of complete muscle paralysis, except for the muscles of the eyes, and this is when dreaming occurs. The sleep cycle refers to these five stages of sleep. It usually takes about ninety minutes to go through the cycle once, starting at stage I and ending at stage V, or REM sleep. After stage V sleep, you return to stage I and repeat the cycle again. On an average night, most people go through the sleep cycle five times. In adults, non-REM sleep predominates at the beginning of the night, only to be gradually replaced by longer and longer periods of REM sleep as morning approaches. It seems that both non-REM and REM sleep are critically important, each in their own way, to the proper functioning of the sleep cycle. It is thought that non-REM sleep is needed to provide time for the brain to repair itself.[3]

During the course of normal activity, the awake brain is thought to accumulate free radicals as byproducts of metabolism. These free radicals, it is postulated, need to be removed before they start damaging healthy nerve cells in the brain, and the time to accomplish this task is provided during non-REM sleep. This may help to explain why smaller animals, with higher metabolic rates, need more time to sleep. In essence, they need more time to deal with the byproducts of their metabolism.[3]

The purpose of REM sleep, on the other hand, has been more difficult for researchers to explain. Since brainwave activity during REM sleep is sometimes greater than that of the awake brain, many scientists think its purpose is more active than passive. If non-REM sleep represents time for the engine to cool down, then REM sleep may be thought to represent time for the engine to be fine-tuned. Indeed, many think REM sleep is critical to the proper development of the brain; they see it as a time when nerve connections are made, and when instinctual behavior becomes more firmly established.

The fact that REM sleep is the predominate sleep of infants and small children only helps to substantiate these claims. When this normal sleep cycle gets disrupted, as is often the case, then major repairs (during non-REM sleep) and major improvements (during REM sleep) to the functioning of the brain fail to get done, leading to a person's body not running very efficiently.

The Sleep Debt—A High Price to Pay

Researchers estimate between 30 and 40 percent of all adults in the United States experience some difficulty with their sleep during a typical year. They also estimate that between 10 and 15 percent of adults have such major problems that they meet the criteria for chronic insomnia, which would be present nearly every night of the year.[4,5]

Many voluntarily become sleep-deprived, while others have such poor sleep habits that insomnia becomes a learned condition. The bottom line is that a large portion of the population is not getting the sleep it needs. Many people are tired, and as a result society must pay a price. Researchers at the National Institutes of Health's National Center for Sleep Disorders Research estimated this price to be about 16 billion dollars in 2003.

On a personal level, sleep deprivation leads to poorer job performance, impaired cognition, and strained intrapersonal relationships. It contributes to decreased immunity against infections, and it frequently precedes bouts of depression and anxiety, suggesting a possible causative role in those. Its involvement in motor vehicle accidents, especially among young adult males, is probably the most tangible of its negative consequences. Studies have shown that sleepy drivers perform as badly as, or worse than, drivers who had been drinking. The National Highway Traffic Safety Administration estimates that over 100,000 accidents a year are the direct result of sleep-deprived drivers.[6,7]

In the last half of the last century, many major world disasters, including the Exxon Valdez oil spill, the nuclear meltdowns at Three Mile Island and Chernobyl, and the Challenger space shuttle explosion, have all been linked to insufficient sleep.[8]

Sleep experts agree that most people should get about eight hours of *quality* sleep a night. When they fall short of that amount, they start accumulating a sleep debt, which has to eventually be paid in order for the body to run properly.

There are many reasons people run up this debt. Stress is one common cause. Affecting nearly everyone, heightened stress leads to predictable responses in the body. Elevations of blood pressure, heart rate, and stress hormones all contribute to a body that's readier for battle than for sleep. This, coupled with the quiet of the night when they lie down to sleep, makes people more likely to think about how to solve their problems than drift into peaceful slumber.

Stress, more than anything, contributes to the development of bad sleep habits. When stressed, people are more inclined to have erratic bedtimes, they are more likely to turn to alcohol to help them fall asleep, and they are more likely to partake in eating binges at night. All these behaviors affect the normal progression of the sleep cycle, and lead to less restorative sleep. When these behaviors become learned, and part of the routine, then people run the risk of letting temporary stressors lead to the development of more chronic sleep problems.

Common Disruptors of Sleep

Sometimes it can be very difficult to discriminate between normal stress, which most people experience, and overwhelming stress, which might be better classified as anxiety. Anxiety, and its counterpart, depression, is incredibly common in society; it is frequently situational and is almost always associated with sleep problems. It is estimated that, for as many as 50 percent of those who have insomnia, depression or anxiety is an underlying condition. In many cases, the insomnia occurs first, sometimes months before the anxiety or depressive symptoms become apparent.[9,10]

Given that the treatment strategies for anxiety and depression are far different than those for insomnia, it is critical to recognize these conditions early. In so doing, you will be focusing on the *cause* rather than the *symptom* of insomnia, and in the long run, you will be much better off.

In addition to depression and anxiety, there are many other medical conditions that can adversely affect a person's sleep. As men get older, their prostate naturally enlarges, leading to incomplete emptying of the bladder and frequent bathroom trips. This repeated interruption of the sleep cycle makes men less likely to have restorative sleep, as they continually have to restart the cycle over from the beginning. Pain, in general, can also lead to disrupted sleep. People with arthritis, back pains, and other orthopedic conditions are much more likely to have fragmented sleep. This, in turn, leads to people with lower pain thresholds, *as less sleep tends to generate more pain.* A vicious cycle results wherein pain disrupts sleep, and disrupted sleep increases pain. Fibromyalgia, a chronic muscle-pain condition where the treatment is dependent on improving the quality of sleep, is a good demonstration of exactly how this relationship works. Aside from pain, almost any chronic medical condition can increase the risk of sleep problems, either directly by affecting breathing, or indirectly through the side effects of drugs. Many of them affect sleep. Some can be sedating, leading to a drugged feeling in the morning, while others can be activating, making it near impossible to fall asleep.

Common Disorders of Sleep

After considering the medical causes and eliminating those related to stress, it is estimated that only 10 percent of the people with insomnia have a primary sleep disorder.[11]

Sleep apnea and restless leg syndrome are two of the more common sleep disorders that many people experience. Sleep apnea, affecting more than 18 million Americans, is characterized by repeated periods during the night when breathing stops. The person's airway gets temporarily obstructed, which results in the stoppage of breathing. People with sleep apnea tend to be obese, they tend to be very loud snorers, and they tend to always be tired. They rarely awaken refreshed, and they frequently fall asleep during the day. Many people fail to comprehend the potential health threat that sleep apnea poses. When there is even the briefest cessation in breathing, oxygen levels in the blood can drop dangerously low, stressing both the brain and the heart. Anyone with chronic sleep apnea, specifically anyone who never gets treated, often complains of headaches and trouble concentrating.

There is also a tendency to develop heart problems. It can be downright scary to watch the heart monitor of someone who has sleep apnea. There are usually skipped beats, fast beats, widened beats, and slow beats. Even an untrained observer can tell that what they are seeing is not normal. What many fail to realize is that sleep apnea can shorten life expectancy considerably. Fortunately, there are treatments, both surgical and medical, that can correct or control the condition. The problem is that many people fail to get diagnosed, or fail to get treated.[12]

Restless leg syndrome is another sleep disorder that frequently flies underneath the radar. It is estimated that more than 12 million Americans are affected. Described by many as an unpleasant sensation in the legs, it is a condition where people have an incredible urge to move their legs in order to get some relief. Thought to be related to a decrease in dopamine, the same hormone involved in Parkinson's disease, restless leg syndrome frequently goes undiagnosed and unappreciated. Its tendency to contribute to fragmented sleep is well-documented. Its real problem lies in its treatment. The idea of starting Parkinson-like medication for a condition that is very annoying, but not disabling, can be intimidating to both doctors and patients alike. If you are someone with this problem, you may first want to try some exercise, such as walking, to see if this may actually help to lessen your discomfort.

When dealing with any of the sleep-disrupting conditions, treatment can be difficult for a variety of reasons. For starters, most people don't seek medical attention until the problem becomes severe. Instead, they chose to self-medicate with alcohol and over-the-counter drugs, which tend to make things worse. It is only after weeks, or sometimes months, of poor sleep that people are forced to find some help. By this time, they are usually desperate to get some relief, and willing to try almost anything to get some restful sleep. If the problem is severe, there are drugs approved by the Food and Drug Administration (FDA) for the short-term treatment of insomnia. But, extreme caution should be used as these drugs can be impairing, especially in older people, and once started, they can be difficult to get off. These should always be used in combination with other strategies directed at treating the primary problem, whether it is stress-related, psychological, or medical.

Home Remedies—Less Sleep, More Caffeine

In addition to self-medicating at night, many people attempt to compensate for their lack of sleep by powering themselves with caffeine in the morning. Many have become so dependent on its ability to increase alertness that they would be in a panic if their access to it were denied. The major question is whether or not this caffeine use is bad for people, and if so, is there a safe limit? It is estimated that more than 80 percent of the world's population ingests caffeine on a daily basis, making it the most consumed drug on the planet. It is primarily found in coffees, teas, chocolates, and sodas. And for those so affected, missing caffeine for just one day can cause withdrawal headaches so severe that most chronic users won't even consider quitting. Americans would be considered moderate consumers on the world scale, consuming on average about 200 milligrams a day. By comparison, some Scandinavian countries average *twice* that amount daily.[13,14]

In the body, caffeine is thought to work by blocking the action of adenosine, an inhibitory hormone, and its effects are primarily stimulating. By increasing mood, energy, and alertness, its perceived effects are extremely positive for the consumer, which further facilitates its continued use. Caffeine generally gets absorbed rapidly from the stomach, and tends to last about six hours. There may be some marginal blood-pressure elevations with caffeine consumption, although some argue that these elevations are more significant after the first cup of coffee in the morning. Whether these effects on blood pressure result in any increase in cardiovascular events is a matter of debate. Most studies seem to conclude that moderate caffeine intake (200–400 milligrams daily) has not been associated with any seriously adverse events. With the advent of the commercial coffee shops and their super strong coffees, however, these conclusions may change.[15]

Carpe Nox—Seize the Night

Fatigue is one of the most common reasons why people come to see me in the office. They usually complain of feeling tired, achy, irritable, and unmotivated. Hoping there may be some medical condition underlying their tiredness, they frequently become disappointed when I shift the attention toward their sleep, or lack of it. This disappointment happens, in large measure, because people don't want to waste more of their time sleeping. They think the answer cannot possibly be that simple, but in most cases, if the sleep becomes corrected, so, too, does the fatigue.

Most people underestimate how much better they feel, and how much better they function, when they are well-rested. When you get sufficient sleep, you become more efficient at work, you think more clearly, you're healthier, and ultimately, you live life happier.

Sleep Tips

1. Value sleep by refusing to voluntarily restrict its time. Most people need about eight to eight and a half hours of sleep a night. When you try to get by with less, you will likely pay the price.

2. Avoid caffeine at least six hours before going to bed. A late afternoon coffee, tea, or soda can seriously affect your ability to sleep hours later. Also, avoid using alcohol as a sleep aid—sleep induced by alcohol tends to bypass the normal sleep cycle, making things worse rather than better.

3. Deal with your stress before you lie down. Stress temporarily disrupts everyone's sleep from time to time. Acknowledging that stress exists is the first step in actually dealing with it. Exercising, venting to friends, and constructive problem-solving are all proven ways to defuse pressure.

4. Try to get more quiet time during the day. In today's world, incessant noise abounds, making silence a novelty only experienced at bedtime. Try to enjoy this treat more during the day and you will sleep more during the night.

5. Develop good sleep hygiene by using the bed for sleeping only. Reading, watching television, and lying awake in bed all contribute to training the body not to fall asleep when it slips underneath the covers.

6. Maximally treat any and all medical conditions that could be disrupting sleep. You should especially consider anxiety and depression potential culprits as they are very common in society. They frequently are linked to sleep problems, and they are very treatable.

7. Seek medical attention if a sleep problem persists. A physician can help you work through the list of possible causes in order to find the best treatment. An untreated sleep condition can negatively impact your health, your mental well-being, and your quality of life.

10

LIVING THE COMMITMENT
TO BETTER HEALTH

I awoke to find myself in a dark woods,
the right path fully lost to me.
—DANTE, *DIVINE COMEDY*

M y wife and I bought our first house in the fall of 1995, shortly
after we were married, when I was in the middle of my resi-
dency training. Money was tight, but we were determined to own
rather than rent. After a seemingly endless search, we settled on a nice
little house that needed some work, but was within our price range.
Seeing the size of my school debt, however, the bank was at first hesitant about approving us for a mortgage, but after some reassurance,
we were granted one, and we were on our way.

Or so we thought. The settlement was a mess. The title company
miscalculated our taxes and we needed several thousand more than we
had in our bank account. The sellers threatened to sue us, our agent
started yelling that we had defaulted on the loan, and my wife and I
felt as though the world had turned against us. But we persevered and
after protracted negotiations, the matter got resolved, and we became
proud homeowners.

When it came time to actually enter the front door of our new
purchase, we experienced another setback. In addition to removing
every light bulb in the house, as a special going away present the sellers had helped themselves to the dining room chandelier, leaving only
open wires hanging from the ceiling. Sitting in the dark on the floor
of our living room, questioning what we had gotten ourselves into, we

started feeling overwhelmed by all that needed to be done. As ill-prepared as we had been for the settlement, we were even less prepared for owning a home. We needed to begin fixing up the house, and we needed to begin right away. The question was where to start.

I learned a lot from that home improvement project—first and foremost, that I didn't know anything about home repairs. My father and my father-in-law became my mentors, showing me how to do things, telling me where to go, and who to ask for help. I tried reading home-improvement books, although I have to admit, it was much easier having someone tell me, show me, or do it for me, than reading about it myself. More than anything else, my father-in-law taught me the value of organization. He always had the perfect tool for the job that needed to be done. His workbench was immaculate, with each piece of equipment neatly resting in its assigned place. His approach to every task was systematic, and he paid special attention to the details.

Most importantly, I learned that my motivation to finish a job was directly related to necessity. If there was a leak in the basement, it became necessary to try and fix it. It demanded my immediate attention, and if it cost a lot of money to hire someone to do it, then it became necessary that I learn how to do it myself.

Your health is much like that house in need of repairs. Without preventive maintenance, it, too, will break down. The same principles effective in fixing the house are also effective in fixing your health. Increasing knowledge, understanding what motivates you, and, above all, getting organized are the foundations on which your health stands. The better you are at developing these foundations, the better your overall health will be.

The question becomes—where does this development begin?

Sooner or Later—All Roads Lead Here

The doctor's office provides the perfect backdrop for the education, motivation, and organization of people in their quest to be healthier. Unfortunately, this tremendous resource often goes untapped. Most people only make appointments to see their doctor when they are sick, or when they have chronic medical conditions. It is estimated that only

20 percent of all office visits to primary care physicians are for the sole purpose of preventive healthcare. Despite this fact, preventive medicine has, more than anything else, been responsible for increasing the life expectancy of Americans. In its series on the Ten Greatest Public Health Achievements, the Centers for Disease Control and Prevention attempted to quantify this impact by reporting that preventive healthcare was responsible for twenty-five out of the thirty-year gain in life expectancy during the previous century.[1,2]

The ultimate goal behind preventive healthcare is to maintain and improve the quality of life, which is primarily achieved by adopting strategies that focus on prevention—not getting sick in the first place— and, barring that, early detection of disease. By promoting healthier lifestyles, it is hoped that the burden of disease on individuals, as well as society, will be lessened.

Surprisingly, prevention or early detection of disease is often easier said than done. Experts, before they are able to issue any recommendations, must take into account a variety of factors. They must be convinced that the disease in question is worth preventing; that there are effective measures to actually prevent it; that the risk of treating the disease preemptively is less than the risk of the disease itself; and that the costs are not prohibitive.

This Just In—Today's Medicine Changes All the Time

Heart disease is a good example of a disease worth preventing. Responsible for more death and disability than most other diseases combined, the impact of heart disease on society is impossible to calculate. Fortunately, though, there are proven ways to lessen its impact. Controlling your cholesterol, improving your blood pressure, lowering your weight, eliminating smoking (if you smoke), and increasing the exercise you do, have all amassed mountains of evidence from clinical trials to show they can reduce the chances of your having a heart attack.

The problem is that new evidence keeps coming in all the time. Since 1990, there have been two revisions in the cholesterol guidelines, three revisions in the blood-pressure guidelines, numerous releases of diet books, and the re-release of an old medication to help

people quit smoking. It's no wonder that people have difficulty staying up-to-date—the speed at which information changes is just too
rapid. In this context, the routine office visit takes on greater and
greater importance. By designating time specifically for health maintenance, you can gain confidence by knowing you are doing everything
possible for the benefit of your health.

Don't Look, Don't Find—
How Cancer Sneaks Up on People

Cancer is a condition well worth preventing. It affects three out of
every four families, placing second only to heart disease in causes of
death, and extracting a mental as well as a physical toll.[3]

A problem arises in actually preventing it, however. While such
behaviors as smoking, excessive drinking, and prolonged sunning
all increase the risk of eventually getting cancer, there is a time disconnect between the behavior and the cancer. People may smoke for
thirty years before getting diagnosed with lung cancer, or they may
worship the sun most of their lives before developing skin cancer.
With such a separation in time between the behavior and the adverse
event, it's no surprise that the threat of cancer doesn't do much to
change most people's behavior. This, coupled with the fact that many
cancers don't have an identifiable cause, has shifted the focus of attention to early detection. Mammograms, pap smears, prostate exams,
and colon checks are all designed to find cancer in its early stages,
when it's theoretically most curable. With improvements in technology, it is getting easier and easier to accomplish this task. Given the
time constraints under which most doctors operate, and given that
most of these screening tests need to get repeated, routine appointments make the most sense in ensuring that what needs to be done,
gets done.

Ready, or Not?

Getting something done, though, involves more than just being told
what to do; it involves being motivated as well. Good physicians,

almost by definition, must be good motivators. They must be able to convince people that they should make changes, and more important, that they *can* make changes. In order to be successful in this task, doctors need to accurately determine a person's *stage of readiness*.

When faced with changing behavior, people predictably go through a series of stages. There is the pre-contemplative stage, when there is no thought of changing behavior; the contemplative stage, when some initial thoughts of changing are entertained; the preparatory stage, when active plans are formulated; the active stage, when those plans are put into action; and the maintenance stage, when the new behavior is reinforced.[4]

Most people passively exist in the pre-contemplative stage, too busy with work and family to seriously consider changing or improving themselves. Everyone, though, has moments of inspiration. Often precipitated by reading a newspaper article, or talking with a friend, people become interested in learning about their health and ways to improve it. It is at this point that they move into the contemplative stage, the critical juncture between possible change or return to the status quo. Those who take the next step and see their doctors to discuss what they may have learned have the best chance of ultimately succeeding in improving themselves. A good office visit is one where people advance their stage of readiness. It is one that gets them from just thinking about change to actually changing. Good doctors are trained to guide people toward healthier lifestyles, and they can follow up on this training by helping their patients develop practical plans.

The true keys to putting theory into practice involve developing a plan, paying attention to detail, and getting organized—this is how to put theory into action. Most people know what they should do, it's the *doing it* that gets them into trouble. Those who are good at organizing themselves are best able to implement these plans.

By having a simple routine, such as always writing things down, keeping a weekly planner, and maintaining a private health file, you can significantly increase your chances of doing everything you should to benefit your health. The use of memory cues can help remind you that certain tests or appointments need to be done. Scheduling all your appointments in the same month, possibly your birthday month, is a good example of this type of memory aid. Enlisting others is also effective in getting things done. Exercising with a friend, going on a diet with a partner, getting healthier together, all are proven ways you can succeed.

For a Good Time, Call . . .

During World War I when the Western Front was a stalemate, morale was low, the countries were war-weary, and the military leaders of the Allies were desperate to get America into the war. When asked just how many soldiers would be needed to tilt the balance in their favor, one astute leader responded, "just one." He reasoned that if America sent just one soldier, it would be making a commitment to the war, and if one came over, many more would follow.

The same principle applies when getting started on health-improvement projects. The difference between getting things done and never getting started may rest on whether someone is able to make just one call. Calling for a doctor's appointment to have a routine checkup represents commitment. It is a tangible act signifying someone's moving from thinking about change to actually changing.

Feel the Force—Creating Positive Energy

My wife is very good at organizing. She balances work, family, and self in such a way that she makes it look easy. One of her secrets is eliminating clutter. Clutter, more than anything else, disrupts well-intended, neatly designed plans. In its attempts to simplify the home, *feng shui* embraces this concept. This ancient Chinese practice stresses the importance of creating open spaces, eliminating unnecessary items, and developing positive energy flow in the form of *chi*.

When you see your doctor for a routine visit, you are, in a sense, trying to remove the clutter from your life. It provides an excellent opportunity to focus on self; it allocates time to consolidate information that you may have learned outside the office; it reminds you about the benefits of exercise and nutrition; and it permits self-assessment enabling you to see where you stand physically, mentally, and emotionally. By taking a proactive approach, you are creating an attitude of positive energy that should lead to a healthier, happier lifestyle.

Getting Started Tips

1. Keep your own health file at home. (Ask for copies of all your test results.)

2. Keep a date book exclusively for your health.

3. Schedule routine office visits. (If you don't know whether your doctor still practices in town, then you've been away too long.)

4. Encourage friends, family, and co-workers to do the first three things listed here. (Try not to be too annoying.)

5. Don't be afraid or embarrassed by colon preps, prostate exams, and mammograms. (These temporary inconveniences could help to avert the more permanent inconvenience of living with cancer.)

6. Take the time to write down your family's medical history. (Similar things tend to break down in the same model of car.)

7. Talk to your kids early and often about the hazards of smoking, the fun of exercise, and the benefits of eating right. (Then back up your talking to them by not smoking, by exercising, and by eating right.)

EPILOGUE

To be healthy, or not to be healthy, that is the question.
Whether 'tis nobler in the mind to live for the day, without
care for tomorrow, suffering the slings and arrows that this
will surely bring, or to take action to plot a different course,
avoiding this sea of trouble, hoping to secure more days
on which to sail upon the water; alas, this is the rub,
live for the day or live more days . . .

Many people approach health with this all-or-none mentality. Too busy with work and family, they spend the bulk of their time taking health for granted, living with little regard for what may be healthy, with behaviors passively on autopilot. Then, provoked by feeling unwell, they get temporarily inspired, reclaiming control of their actions, becoming engrossed in everything healthy, only to be eventually distracted by life again. Like a broken record, this pattern continually repeats itself, resulting in the gradual deterioration of health, and over time making people more and more dependent on a healthcare system that itself is in desperate need of repair.

In many ways, healthcare now could be described as being in its *best of times* and *worst of times*. Through advancements in technology, increased specialization of doctors and improvements in medicine, the quality of healthcare has never been better. Problems, however, start to arise when it comes to paying for the advanced technology, dealing with the enlarged bureaucracy, and affording the improved medicines.

By empowering yourself with knowledge about the basics of being healthy, you will become a little less reliant on a healthcare delivery system that is obviously flawed.

This knowledge base will only be developed when people start valuing their health. Health is wealth; it is the currency that allows you to do anything your heart desires. It is at the core of your freedom, at the core of your happiness, and at the core of your family life. When people start seeing health as valuable, then and only then, will everyone become interested in learning ways to actually improve it.

Recalled to Health is intended to start this learning process. Its goals are primarily directed toward motivating, educating, and organizing you in your quest to be healthier. If it accomplishes little more than making you think seriously about your health, then it can be considered a success.

The concept of being recalled is less about being an epiphany and more about being an affirmation. It's not about you suddenly seeing the light, but rather it's about you consistently making the commitment, day after day, week after week, to follow healthier behaviors. Most of you can do this temporarily, but then get easily distracted by the fast-paced world. When you get too far off course, you need to be reminded; and when you start taking your greatest asset for granted, you need to be *recalled*.

In memory of
William Hennessy
1929–2009

Love you, Dad.

References

Chapter 4

1. Rosenson, RS, Otvos, JD, Freedman, DS. "Relations of lipoprotein subclass levels and low-density size to progression of coronary artery disease in the Pravastatin Limitation of Atherosclerosis in the Coronary Arteries (PLAC-1) Trial." *American Journal of Cardiology* 90:89, 2002.

2. Nishimura, RA. "Cardiology Part IV." *Mayo Clinic Internal Medicine Board Review 2002–2003:* 96–97.

3. Lipid Research Clinics Program. "The Lipid Research Clinics Coronary Primary Prevention Trial results, II: the relationship of reduction in incidence of coronary heart disease to cholesterol lowering." *Journal of the American Medical Association* 251:365–374, 1984.

4. Shepherd, J, Cobbe, SM, Ford, I, et al. "Prevention of coronary heart disease with pravastatin in men with hypercholesterolemia." *New England Journal of Medicine* 333:1301, 1995.

5. Sacks, FM, Pfeffer, MA, Moye, LA, et al. for the Cholesterol and Recurrent Events Trial investigators. "The effect of pravastatin on coronary events after myocardial infarction in patients with average cholesterol levels." *New England Journal of Medicine* 335:1001, 1996.

6. LIPID Study Group. "The Long-term Intervention with Pravastatin in Ischemic Heart Disease (LIPID) Study Group: prevention of cardiovascular events and death with pravastatin in patients with coronary artery disease and a broad range of initial cholesterol levels." *New England Journal of Medicine* 339:1357, 1998.

7. Scandinavian Simvastatin Survival Study Group. "Randomized trial of cholesterol lowering in 4444 patients with coronary artery disease: the Scandinavian Simvastatin Survival Study (4S)." *The Lancet* 344:1383, 1994.

8. Chien, PC, Frishman, WH. "Lipid Disorders." In *Current Diagnosis and Treatment in Cardiology* (2nd ed) edited by MH Crawford. New York: McGraw-Hill, 2003.

9. National Cholesterol Education Program Expert Panel. "Executive summary of the third report of the National Cholesterol Education Program (NCEP) expert panel on detection, evaluation, and treatment of high blood cholesterol in adults (Adult Treatment Panel III)." *Journal of the American Medical Association* 285:2486, 2001.

10. Grundy, SM, Cleeman, JI, et al. "Implications of recent clinical trials for the National Cholesterol Education Program Adult Treatment Panel III guidelines." *Circulation* 110:227–239, 2004.

Chapter 5

1. Pate, RR, Pratt, M, Blair, SN, et al." Physical activity and public health: a recommendation from the Centers for Disease Control and Prevention and the American College of Sports Medicine." *Journal of the American Medical Association* 273:402–407, 1995.

2. Caspersen, CJ, Powell, KE, Christenson, GM. "Physical activity, exercise, and physical fitness: definitions and distinctions for health-related research." *Public Health Report* 100:126–131, 1985.

3. Thompson, PD, Buchner, D, et al. "Exercise and physical activity in the prevention and treatment of atherosclerotic cardiovascular disease." *Circulation* 107:3109–3116, 2003.

4. Blair, SN, Jackson, AS. "Physical fitness and activity as separate heart disease risk factors: a meta-analysis." *Medicine & Science in Sports & Exercise* 33:762–764, 2001.

5. O'Connor, GT, Buring, JE, Yusuf, S, et al. "An overview of randomized trials of rehabilitation with exercise after myocardial infarction." *Circulation* 80:234–244, 1989.

6. Paffenbarger, RS, Hyde, RT, Wing, AL, et al. "Physical activity, all-cause mortality, and longevity of college alumni." *New England Journal of Medicine* 314: 605–613, 1986.

7. See note 1 above.

8. Wing, RR, Hill, JO. "Successful weight loss maintenance." *Annual Review of Nutrition* 21:323–341, 2001.

9. Fagard, RH. "Exercise characteristics and the blood pressure response to dynamic physical training." *Medicine & Science in Sports & Exercise* 33:S484–492, 2001.

10. Knowler, WC, Barrett-Connor, E, Fowler, SE, et al. for the Diabetes Prevention Program Research Group. "Reduction in the incidence of type 2 diabetes with lifestyle intervention or metformin." *New England Journal of Medicine* 346:393–403, 2002.

11. Pollock, KM. "Exercise in treating depression: broadening the psychotherapist's role." *Journal of Clinical Psychology* 57:1289–1300, 2001.

12. Vuori, IM. "Dose-response of physical activity and low back pain, osteoarthritis, and osteoporosis." *Medicine & Science in Sports & Exercise* 33:S551–586, 2001.

13. Breslow, RA, Ballard-Barbash, R, Munoz, K, et al. "Long-term recreational physical activity and breast cancer in the National Health and Nutrition Examination Survey I epidemiologic follow-up study." *Cancer Epidemiology, Biomarkers and Prevention* 10:805–808, 2001.

14. Slattery, ML, Potter, JD. "Physical activity and colon cancer: confounding or interaction?" *Medicine & Science in Sports & Exercise* 34:913–919, 2002.

15. See note 1 above.

16. King, AC, Sallis, JF, Dunn, AL, et al. for the Activity Counseling Trial Research Group. "Overview of the Activity Counseling Trial (ACT) intervention for promoting physical activity in primary health care settings." *Medicine & Science in Sports & Exercise* 30:1086–1096, 1998.

17. See note 16 above.

18. Thompson, PD, Funk, EJ, Carleton, RA, et al. "Incidence of death during jogging in Rhode Island from 1975 through 1980." *Journal of the American Medical Association* 247:2535–2538, 1982.

Chapter 6

1. National High Blood Pressure Education Program Coordinating Committee. "The seventh report of the Joint National Committee on prevention, detection, evaluation, and treatment of high blood pressure: the JNC VII report." *Journal of the American Medical Association* 289:2560–2572, 2003.

2. Lewington, S, Clarke, R, Qizilbash, N, et al. "Age-specific relevance of usual blood pressure to vascular mortality." *The Lancet* 360:1903–1913, 2002.

3. Yarrows, S, Julius, S, Pickering, T. "Home blood pressure monitoring." *Archives of Internal Medicine* 160:1251–1257, 2000.

4. Crenner, CW. "Introduction of the blood pressure cuff into U.S. medical practice: technology and skilled practice." *Annals of Internal Medicine* 128:488–493, 1998.

5. Lewis, C. "Checking up on blood pressure monitors." *FDA Consumer* 10–11, Sept–Oct 2002.

6. Bailey, RH, Knaus, VL, Bauer, JH. "Aneroid sphygmomanometers: an assessment of accuracy at a university hospital and clinics." *Archives of Internal Medicine* 151:1409–1412, 1991.

7. ANSI/AAMI SP10–1987, et al. "American national standard for electronic or automated sphygmomanometers"; http://www.ami.org/standards.

8. O'Brien, E, Petrie, J, Littler, WA, et al. "The British Hypertension Society protocol for the evaluation of blood pressure measuring devices." *Journal of Hypertension* 11(Suppl 2):S43–63, 1993.

9. Pickering, TG, James, GD, Boddie, C, et al. " How common is white coat hypertension?" *Journal of the American Medical Association* 259:225–228, 1988.

10. Ayman, D, Goldshine, AD. "Blood pressure determinations by patients with essential hypertension, I: the difference between clinic and home readings before treatment." *The American Journal of the Medical Sciences* 200:465–474, 1940.

11. Mancia, G, Zanchetti, A, Agebeti-Rosie, E, et al. "Ambulatory blood pressure is superior to clinic blood pressure in predicting treatment-induced regression of left ventricular hypertrophy." *Circulation* 95:1464–1470, 1997.

12. Gosse, P, Promax, H, Durandet, P, et al. " 'White coat' hypertension: no harm for the heart." *Hypertension* 22:766–777, 1993.

13. Palatini, P, Mormini, P, Santonastaso, M, et al, for the HARVEST Study Investigators. "Target organ damage in stage I hypertensive subjects with white coat and sustained hypertension: results from the HARVEST Study." *Hypertension* 31:57–63, 1998.

14. He, J, Whelton, PK, Appel, LJ, et al. "Long-term effects of weight loss and dietary sodium reduction on incidence of hypertension." *Hypertension* 35:544–549, 2000.

15. Cushman, WC, Ford, CE, Culter, JA, et al. "Success and predictors of blood pressure control in diverse North American settings: The Antihypertensive and Lipid-Lowering Treatment to Prevent Heart Attack Trial (ALLHAT)." *Journal of Clinical Hypertension* (*Greenwich*) 4:393–404, 2002.

16. See note 1 above.

17. Neal, B, MacMahon, S, Chapman, N. "Effects of ACE Inhibitors, calcium antagonists, and other blood-pressure-lowering drugs." *The Lancet* 356:1955–1964, 2000.

18. Vasan, RS, Beiser, A, Seshadri, S, et al. "Residual lifetime risk for developing hypertension in middle-aged women and men: the Framingham Heart Study." *Journal of the American Medical Association* 287:1003–1010, 2002.

Websites

1. British Hypertension Society: Blood pressure monitor reviews. Available at: http://www.bhsoc.org/blood_pressure_list.stm

2. Medication reviews. Available at http://www.PDR.net.

Chapter 7

1. Conibear, H. "World consumption trends." *Alcohol in Moderation (AIM) Online Digest* Editorial, March 2005.

2. Rehm, JT, Bondy, SJ, Sempos, CT, et al. "Alcohol consumption and coronary heart disease morbidity and mortality." *American Journal of Epidemiology* 146:495–501, 1997.

3. Klatsky, AL, Armstrong, MA, Friedman, GD. "Red wine, white wine, liquor, beer, and risk for coronary artery disease hospitalization." *American Journal of Cardiology* 80:416–420, 1997.

4. Ajani, UA, Hennekens, CH, Spelsberg, A, et al. "Alcohol consumption and risk of type 2 diabetes mellitus among U.S. male physicians." *Archives of Internal Medicine* 160:1025–1030, 2000.

5. Galanis, DJ, Joseph, C, Masaki, KH, et al. "A longitudinal study of drinking and cognitive performance in elderly Japanese American men: the Honolulu-Asia aging study." *American Journal of Public Health* 90:1254–1259, 2000.

6. Baur, JA, Pearson, KJ, Price, NL, et al. "Resveratrol improves health and survival of mice on high-calorie diet." *Nature* 444:337–342, Nov 2006.

7. Goldberg, DM, Yan, J, Soleas, GJ. "Absorption of three wine-related polyphenols in three different matrices by healthy subjects." *Clinical Biochemistry* 36:79–87, 2003.

8. Corder, R, et al. "Oenology: Red wine procyanidins and vascular health." *Nature* 444:566, Nov 2006.

9. Bayard, V, Chamorro, F, Motta, J, et al. "Does flavonol intake influence mortality from nitric oxide-dependent processes? Ischemic heart disease, stroke, diabetes mellitus, and cancer in Panama." *International Journal of Medical Science* 4(1):53–58, 2007.

10. Taubert, D, Roesen, R, Lehmann, C, et al. "Effects of low habitual cocoa intake on blood pressure and bioactive nitric oxide: a randomized controlled trial. *Journal of the American Medical Association* 298:49–60, 2007.

11. Hollenberg, NK. "Heart-healthy compound in chocolate identified." *ScienceDaily* January 20, 2006; http://www.sciencedaily.com.

12. Bang, HO, Dyerberg, J. "The composition of food consumed by Greenlandic Eskimos." *Acta Medica Scandunavia* 200:69–73, 1973.

13. Hibbeln, JR. "Healthy intakes of n–3 and n–6 fatty acids: estimates considering worldwide diversity." *American Journal of Clinical Nutrition* 83(6 Supplement): 1483S–1493S, 2006.

14. Simopoulos, AP. "The importance of the ratio of omega-6/omega-3 essential fatty acids." *Biomedicine & Pharmacotherapy* 56(8):365–379, Oct 2002.

15. Kris-Etherton, PM, Harris, WS, Appel, LJ. "Fish consumption, fish oil, omega-3 fatty acids, and cardiovascular disease." *Circulation* 106(21):2747–2757, 2002.

16. Connor, WE. "Importance of *n*–fatty acids in health and disease." *American Journal of Clinical Nutrition* 71(1 Supplement):171S–175S, 2000.

17. Brouwer, IA, Katan, MB, Zock, PL. "Dietary alpha-linolenic acid is associated with reduced risk of fatal coronary heart disease, but increased prostate cancer risk: a meta-analysis." *Journal of Nutrition* 134(4):919–922, 2004.

18. Bucher, HC, Hengstler, P, Schindler, C, et al. "*n*–3 polyunsaturated fatty acids in coronary heart disease: a meta-analysis of randomized controlled trials." *The American Journal of Medicine* 112(4):298–304, 2002.

19. Burr, ML, Sweetham, PM, Fehily, AM. "Diet and reinfarction." *European Heart Journal* 15(8):1152–1153, 1994.

20. Stone, NJ. "Fish consumption, fish oil, lipids, and coronary heart disease." *Circulation* 94:2337–2340, 1996.

21. The GISSI Study Group. "Dietary supplementation with *n*–3 polyunsaturated fatty acids and vitamin E after myocardial infarction: results of the GISSI-Prevenzione trial." *The Lancet* 354:447–455, 1999.

22. Harris, WS. "N-3 fatty acids and serum lipoproteins: human studies." *American Journal of Clinical Nutrition* 65(5 Supplement):1645S–1654S, 1997.

23. Sumpio, BE, Cordova, AC, et al. "Green tea, the *Asian paradox*, and cardiovascular disease." *Journal of the American College of Surgeons* 202:813–825, 2006.

24. Imai, K, Nakachi, K. "Cross sectional study effects of drinking green tea on cardiovascular and liver diseases." *British Medical Journal* 310:693, 1995.

25. Peters, U, Poole, C, Arab, L. "Does tea affect cardiovascular disease? A meta-analysis. *American Journal of Epidemiology* 15:495–503, 2001.

26. Mukamal, KJ, Maclure, M, Muller, JE, et al. "Tea consumption and mortality after acute myocardial infarction." *Circulation* 105:E9109–E9110, 2002.

27. Wakai, K, Ohno, Y, Obata, K. "Prognostic significance of selected lifestyle factors in urinary bladder cancer." *Japanese Journal of Cancer Research* 84:1223–1229, 1993.

28. Bushman, JL. "Green tea and cancer in humans: a review of the literature." *Nutrition and Cancer: An International Journal* 31:151–159, 1998.

29. Zhang, M, Binns, CW, Lee, AH. "Tea consumption and ovarian cancer risk: a case-control study in China." *Cancer Epidemiology Biomarkers & Prevention* 11:713–718, 2002.

30. Setiawan, VW, Zhang, ZF, Yu, GP, et al. "Protective effect of green tea on the risks of chronic gastritis and stomach cancer." *International Journal of Cancer* 92:600–604, 2001.

31. Seely, D, Mills, EJ, Wu, P, et al. "The effects of green tea consumption on incidence of breast cancer and recurrence of breast cancer: a systematic review and meta-analysis." *Integrative Cancer Therapy* 4:144–155, 2005.

32. Bernstein, BJ, Grasso, T. "Prevalence of complementary and alternative medicine use in cancer patients." *Oncology* 15:1267–1272, 2001.

Chapter 8

1. Flegal, KM, Carro, MD, Ogden, CL, et al. "Prevalence and trends in obesity among U.S. adults, 1999–2000." *Journal of the American Medical Association* 288:1723–1727, 2002.

2. Satcher, D. "The Surgeon General's call to action to prevent and decrease overweight and obesity." U.S. Department of Health and Human Services, Public Health Services, Office of the Surgeon General, 2001; http://www.surgeongeneral.gov/topics/obesity.

3. Rand, CS, Macgregor, AM. "Successful weight loss following obesity surgery and the perceived liability of morbid obesity." *International Journal of Obesity* 15: 577–579, 1991.

4. Spake, A."Hey, maybe it's not a weakness. Just maybe...it's a disease." *US. News & World Report* 51–56, Feb 9, 2004.

5. Cummings, DE, Shannon, MH. "Roles for ghrelin in the regulation of appetite and body weight." *Archives of Surgery* 138:389–396, 2003.

6. Hansen, TK, Dall, R, Hosoda, H, et al. "Weight loss increases circulating levels of ghrelin in human obesity." *Clinical Endocrinology (Oxford)*. 56:203–206, 2002.

7. Batterham, RL, Cohen, MA, Ellis, SM, et al. "Inhibition of food intake in obese subjects by peptide YY3–36." *New England Journal of Medicine* 349(10):926–928, Sept 4, 2003.

8. Aziz, A, Anderson, H. "Exendin-4, a GLP-1 receptor agonist, interacts with proteins and their products of digestion to suppress food intake in rats." *Journal of Nutrition* 133(7):2326–2330, 2003.

9. Friedman, JM, Halaas, JL. "Leptin and the regulation of body weight in mammals." *Nature* 395:763–770, 1998.

10. Calvadini, C, Siega-Riz, AM, Popkin, BM. "U.S. adolescent food intake trends from 1965 to 1996." *Archives of Disease in Childhood* 83:18–24, 2000.

11. Bellisle, F, Rolland-Cachera, MF. "How sugar-containing drinks might increase adiposity in children." *The Lancet* 357:490–491, 2001.

12. Nestle, M. "Soft drink 'pouring rights': marketing empty calories to children." *Public Health Report* 115:308–319, 2000.

13. Center for Commercial-Free Public Education. Available at: http://www.preventioninstitute.org, Sept 21, 2002.

14. Young, L, Nestle, M. "The contribution of expanding portion sizes to the U.S. obesity epidemic." *American Journal of Public Health* 92:246–249, Feb 2002.

15. Nielson, SJ, Popkin, BM. "Patterns and trends in food portion sizes, 1977–1998." *Journal of the American Medical Association* 289:450–453, Jan 2003.

16. *Dietary intake data from the Continuing Survey of Food Intakes by Individuals, 1994–1996, Diet and Health Knowledge Survey.* Washington, DC: U.S. Dept. of Agriculture, Dec 1997.

17. *U.S. Trends in Eating Away From Home, 1982–1989* (Statistical Bulletin 926). Washington, DC: U.S. Dept. Agriculture/Economic Research Service, 1995.

18. Clauson, A. "Share of food spending for eating out reaches 47 percent." *Food Review* 22:20–22, 1999.

19. *Food Spending in American Households, 2003–2004* (Economic Information Bulletin No. EIB-23), Washington, DC: U.S. Dept of Agriculture/Economic Research Service, Mar 2007.

20. Hu, FB. "The Mediterranean diet and mortality–olive oil and beyond." *New England Journal of Medicine* 348:2595–2596, 2003.

21. de Lorgeril, M, Salen, P, Martin, JL, et al. *Mediterranean diet, traditional risk factors, and the rate of cardiovascular complications after myocardial infarction: final report of the Lyon Diet Heart Study. Circulation* 99:779–785, 1999.

22. Burr, ML, Gilbert, JH, Holliday, RM, et al. "Effects of changes in fat, fish, and fiber intake on death and myocardial reinfarction: diet and reinfarction trial (DART)." *The Lancet* 2:757–761, 1989.

23. GISSI-Prevenzione Investigators. "Dietary supplementation with n–3 polyunsaturated fatty acids and vitamin E after myocardial infarction: results of the GISSI-Prevenzione trial." *The Lancet* 354:447–455, 1999.

24. Atkins, RC. *Dr. Atkins' New Diet Revolution* New York, NY: Avon Books, 2002.

25. Bravata, DM, Sander, L, Huang, J, et al. "Efficacy and safety of low carbohydrate diets: a systemic review." *Journal of the American Medical Association* 289:1837–1850, 2003.

26. Westman, EC, Yancy, WS, Edman, JS, et al. "Effect of 6-month adherence to a very low carbohydrate diet program." *The American Journal of Medicine* 113:30–36, 2002.

27. Samaha, FF, Iqbal, N, Seshadri, P, et al. "A low-carbohydrate as compared with a low-fat diet in severe obesity." *New England Journal of Medicine* 348:2074–2081, 2003.

28. Brehm, BJ, Seeley, RJ, Daniels, SR, et al. "A randomized trial comparing a very low-carbohydrate diet and a calorie-restricted low-fat diet on body weight and cardiovascular risk factors in healthy women." *Journal of Clinical Endocrinology & Metabolism* 88:1617–1623, 2003.

29. St. Jeor, ST, Howard, BV, Prewitt, TE, et al." Dietary protein and weight reduction: a statement for healthcare professionals from the nutrition committee of the Council on Nutrition, Physical Activity, and Metabolism of the American Heart Association." *Circulation* 104:1869–1874, 2001.

30. Agatston, A. *The South Beach Diet.* Emmaus, PA: Rodale Books, 2003.

Chapter 9

1. Berger, H. "Ueber das elektroenkephalogramm des menschen." *Archiv für Psychiatrie und Nervenkrankheiten* 87:527–570, 1929.

2. Aserinsky, E, Kleitman, N. "Regularly occurring periods of eye motility, and concomitant phenomena." *Science* 118:273–274, 1953.

3. Siegel, JM. "Why we sleep." *Scientific American* 289:92–98, 2003.

4. Mellinger, GD, Balter, MB, Uhlenhuth, EH. "Insomnia and its treatment: prevalence and correlates." *Archives of General Psychiatry* 42(3):225–232, Mar 1985.

5. Lee-Chiong, TL. "Sleep and sleep disorders: an overview." *Medical Clinics of North America* 88, 2004.

6. Pack, AI, Pack, AM, Rodgman, E, et al. "Characteristics of crashes attributed to the driver having fallen asleep." *Accident Analysis & Prevention* 27:769–775, 1995.

7. "Understanding sleep: brain basics." National Institute of Neurological Disorders and Stroke (NINDS)/National Institutes of Health. May 2007. http://www.ninds.nih.gov/disorders/brain_basics/understanding_sleep.htm.

8. Angier, N. "Eye-opener about sleep." *Readers Digest* 139;83:57–59, 1991.

9. Weilburg, JB. "Approach to the patient with insomnia." In *Primary Care Medicine: Office Evaluation and Management of the Adult Patient* (3rd ed) edited by AH Goroll, A Lawrence. Philadelphia, PA: J.B. Lippincott Company, 1995.

10. Nowell, PD, Buysse, DJ. "Treatment of insomnia in patients with mood disorders." *Depression and Anxiety* 14:7–18, 2001.

11. See note 9 above.

12. See note 7 above.

13. James, JE. *Understanding Caffeine: A Biobehavioral Analysis.* Thousand Oaks, CA: Sage Publications, 1997.

14. Fredholm, BB, Battig, K, Holmen, J, et al. "Actions of caffeine in the brain with special reference to factors that contribute to its widespread use." *Pharmacological Reviews* 51:83–133, 1999.

15. Suleman, A, Chawla, J. "Neurologic effects of caffeine"; http://emedicine.medscape.com/article/1182710-overview.

Chapter 10

1. Woodwell, DA, Cherry, DK. "National Ambulatory Medical Care Survey: 2002 Summary." *Advance Data* 346:1–44, 2004.

2. Centers for Disease Control and Prevention. "Ten Greatest Public Health Achievements–United States, 1990–1999." *Morbidity and Mortality Weekly Report* 48: 241–243, 19.

3. Morse, MR, Heffron, WA. *Preventative Health Care: Textbook of Family Practice* (6th ed). Philadelphia, PA: W.B. Saunders, 2002.

4. Prochaska, JO, DiClemente, CC. "Stages of change in the modification of problem behaviors" In *Progress in Behavior Modification Sycamore Press* edited by M Hersen, RM Eisler, and PM Miller. Sycamore, IL: Sycamore Press, 1994.

INDEX

LDL. *See* Lipoproteins, high-density
  (LDL).
Leadership, 21
Legs, 126–127
Leptin, 103–104
Life expectancy, 2
Lipid Research Clinics Coronary Primary
  Prevention Trial, 44
Lipids. *See* Lipoproteins.
Lipoproteins, 41–42
  chylomicrons, 41
  high-density (HDL), 41, 42, 49, 54
  intermediate-density (IDL), 41
  low-density (LDL), 41, 42, 48–49, 50,
    54, 82, 93
  size of, 42–43, 54
  very-low-density (VLDL), 41
  See also Cholesterol.
Lists, daily, 30–31
Liver, 50
Long-Term Intervention with Pravastatin
  in Ischemic Disease (LIPID), 45

Manometers. *See* Blood pressure
  monitors.
McGinley, Edward, 54
Meals, 108–109, 116
Medical history, family, 137
Medical profession, 132–134
Medications
  anti-inflammatory, 78
  blood pressure, 75–76, 78
  cholesterol, 45–46, 50–51, 52–53
  over-the-counter, 71
  sleep, 127
Memory aids, 32–33, 135–136, 137
Metabolism, 61, 111, 112, 123
Moods, 56
Motivations, 7, 16–18, 21, 23, 31, 38, 62,
  134–135
Mulberries, 83

National Center for Sleep Disorders, 124
National Cholesterol Education Program
  (NCEP), 44–45, 46, 49

National Health and Nutrition
  Examination Survey (SHANES), 2
National High Blood Pressure Education
  Program (NHBPEP), 74
National Highway Traffic Safety
  Administration, 124
National Institutes of Health (NIH), 44,
  46
National Weight Control Registry
  (NWCR), 59
NCEP. *See* National Cholesterol
  Education Program (NCEP).
Nitric oxide, 84, 86
Noise, 129
Nuclear magnetic resonance (NMR),
  41–42

Obesity, 99–101
  See also Weight.
Organization, 135–137
Osteoporosis, 60
Oxygen, 42, 69, 82, 126

Pain, 125
Paradoxes, 94
  Asian, 92
  French, 80, 83
Patton, George S., 64
Peanuts, 83
Peptide YY, 103, 104
Peripheral resistance, 70
Physical activity, 7, 31–32, 43, 49, 54,
  55–66, 75, 112, 127, 133, 137
  accumulation of, 58, 65
  aerobic, 78
  commitment to, 64–65, 66, 137
  counseling and, 62–63
  men and, 62–63
  time and, 60–61
  support for, 64, 66, 136
  women and, 62–63
Physical fitness, 117
Pinot Noir, 82–83, 94
Plaque, 41, 42–44, 50, 51–52, 84, 93
Polyphenols, 81–83, 91, 94

About the Author

Timothy J. Hennessy, M.D, is a board-certified internist in a Wilmington, Delaware group practice of primary care physicians. In January 2007, he began writing a health newsletter: *H-mail: Medical Education Made Easy*, which he distributes via e-mail on a bimonthly basis, and which became the initial impetus for writing *Recalled to Health*. This book serves two purposes—it is both a personal memoir detailing his learning experiences on the path to medicine, and a useful medical guide to attaining and maintaining good health.

In addition to his busy practice and his newsletter, Dr. Hennessy, who describes himself as conservative with medicine, is a clinical associate professor of medicine on the teaching faculty of Jefferson Medical College, Philadelphia, Pennsylvania, where he also received his medical degree. He is a board member of the Delaware Academy of Medicine and is the current chairman of the Academy's library system.

His other interests include coaching (soccer and basketball) and reading—his favorite topics include history, autobiographies, and self-improvement. Dr. Tim lives with his wife and three children in Drexel Hill, Pennsylvania. He can be contacted through his website: www.recalledtohealth.com.